CRISIS AT THE FRONT LINE

A Twentieth Century Fund Paper

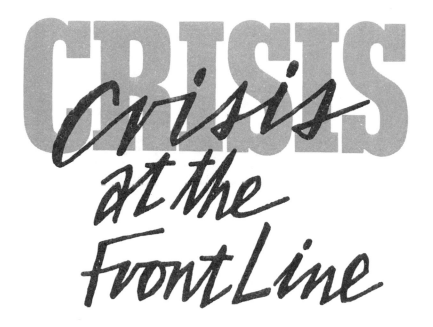

CRISIS

The Effects of AIDS on Public Hospitals

by Dennis P. Andrulis

PP Priority Press Publications/New York/1989

The Twentieth Century Fund is a research foundation undertaking timely analyses of economic, political, and social issues. Not-for-profit and nonpartisan, the Fund was founded in 1919 and endowed by Edward A. Filene.

Library of Congress Cataloging-in-Publication Data
Andrulis, Dennis P.
  Crisis at the front line.

  "A Twentieth Century Fund paper."
  1. AIDS (Disease)—Patients—Hospital care—United
States. 2. Hospitals—United States. 3. AIDS (Disease)
—Government policy—United States. I. Title.
RA644.A25A53   1989   362.1'969792'00973   89-10829
ISBN 0-87078-267-3
ISBN 0-87078-266-5 (pbk.)

Foreword

Public hospitals are distinguished by the sheer volume of the care they provide, the major role they play in the education of physicians and other health care workers, and their ability to provide such vital, yet unprofitable, services as trauma centers. What distinguishes them further is their commitment to serving people without regard to their ability to pay—and the clients they are serving today are drawn from a population as varied as it is growing.

Contrary to the conventional wisdom, a large number of those who cannot pay are workers—those who are catastrophically ill, underinsured, uninsured employees of small businesses or part-time employees, and insured individuals whose preexisting conditions are not covered— and the dependents of all of these groups. In addition, there are the unemployed who have no health insurance; the poor who do not qualify for Medicaid; and drug users, prostitutes, and the homeless. Finally, there are the AIDS victims.

A great deal of attention has been given the impact of the AIDS epidemic on our nation's public hospitals—the strain on the medical staff, the appropriateness of care, and perhaps most important, the drain on their fiscal health. But as Dennis Andrulis, president of the National Public Health and Hospital Institute, persuasively argues in the following pages, the AIDS epidemic does not present us with a new policy problem—instead, it has exposed many of the fundamental flaws in our national approach to health care.

Rather than settling for patchwork measures, Andrulis urges a basic restructuring of the system. Central to that restructuring is a new system of financing. For example, in order to ensure fair and equitable coverage of inpatient and outpatient care, he would have the states, in cooperation with the federal government, guarantee a minimal national level of Medicaid reimbursement in order to relieve the disproportionate burden our current health crises are putting on public hospitals.

But perhaps the most important thing he has done in this examination of public hospitals is to broaden the terms of the policy debate. By using AIDS as a tool with which to examine the structure of the nation's health care system, Dennis Andrulis has shown us the way to improve the lot of all the nation's medically indigent. We are grateful to him for it.

Marcia Bystryn, ACTING DIRECTOR
The Twentieth Century Fund
August 1989

Contents

Dedication

To the administrators and staff at the institutions who are members of the National Association of Public Hospitals. Without their insights and assistance over the years, this project would not have been possible.

Acknowledgments

I would like to thank the many individuals who made this project possible. I would especially like to acknowledge the assistance of Virginia Beers Weslowski, who analyzed public hospital AIDS data and who provided the description of AIDS care in these institutions based on that information.

I would also like to thank Pam Bradley and Debbie Bauer of the National Association of Public Hospitals (NAPH) for their help in preparation of this report. I would also like to acknowledge Elizabeth Hintz and Audrey Spolarich of the National Public Health and Hospital Institute for their assistance in manuscript reviews and Larry Gage at NAPH for his support.

I would like to express my appreciation to my program officer at the Twentieth Century Fund, Jane Hughes, for her guidance and her patience. Special recognition also goes to the tireless efforts of Tammy Mitchell and Beverly Goldberg, for their comments and overall assistance on editing this manuscript.

Chapter 1
Introduction

The AIDS epidemic came on the scene at a time when public hospitals were already facing many critical issues, including high occupancy rates, increases in the numbers of the medically indigent, cost-containment efforts, and serious problems of funding—in particular, reduced capacity of local governments to finance health care services. Acquired Immune Deficiency Syndrome (AIDS) has served to exacerbate each of these issues, while adding significantly to the financial and operational problems already facing the nation's public hospitals.

The following "portraits" reveal much about the problems facing our public hospital system today:

James, age thirty-four, single, and living in a southern city, was diagnosed with AIDS a year ago. For the first months after the diagnosis he was able to continue to work as a computer programmer at a large technology firm. However, his illness exhausted him and caused him to use all available sick leave and vacation time. As a result, he had to resign his position. Now he spends most of his time at home or in the health care system.

Since contracting AIDS, James has been hospitalized twice for opportunistic infections, for ten days each time. His zidovudine (AZT) treatments, while effective in slowing the progress of the disease, had to be stopped due to dangerous side effects. He has been visited at home by volunteers from a local, community-based support group and by a visiting nurse.

His initial stay in the hospital, which cost more than $8,000, was covered by his private insurance as was his expensive AZT therapy. For four months after he resigned from his job, he was able to continue his individual policy, but then he exhausted his personal resources. Although most of his Social Security disability payments and other funds were used for medical purposes, his state's Medicaid program would not qualify him for medical benefits. When he needed his second hospitalization and returned to the private hospital that treated him the first time, he was told they would no longer treat him since he could not pay. A physician at that institution told him to try the public hospital.

The public institution has since assumed responsibility for his treatment. It has also admitted several of his friends, in similar circumstances, to its inpatient unit. The costs of his care, about $8,000 per inpatient stay for hospital and physicians' services, are being absorbed by the institution. The hospital hopes that the county will pay for a large portion of the cost for James's and other similar cases, but its request for additional AIDS assistance for its medically indigent cases, double in 1988 what it was in 1986, has met with increasing resistance. Already, there is talk among the county legislators about their inability to cover the costs of any drugs for AIDS that are as expensive as AZT. Meanwhile, James, who is now at home, wonders whether he will survive his next major AIDS-related infection.

Joanne, a thirty-seven-year-old single New York City native, has been addicted to heroin for ten years. Diagnosed as an AIDS case six months ago, she has been ill continually. Her inability to hold a job for the past ten years has left Joanne dependent on panhandling, petty theft, prostitution, or the public sector. Now she has been admitted to a public hospital with a diagnosis of AIDS-related pneumonia, but she is also suffering from several other conditions that stem from years and years of drug use. At the moment, Joanne remains an inpatient after twenty days for treatments that required acute care hospitalization for seventeen days. Since there is a four-month waiting list for community-based residential care beds and she has no place else to go, the hospital staff has decided to maintain Joanne in the hospital as medically ready to leave the hospital but with no placement available.

Medicaid in New York State will cover much of Joanne's inpatient costs, but the hospital still loses money because she requires such a long stay. In addition, this particular public institution is almost at 100 percent of capacity. The hospital crowding is attributable in part to AIDS, but it also involves many other patient populations such as substance abusers, psychiatric patients, and low-income patients in general. With alternative settings virtually nonexistent, and with sources of financial support for other medical care so meager, the hospital administration and medical personnel wonder what will happen when the epidemic worsens. Joanne wonders whether she will ever leave the hospital alive.

Debra is eight months old. She suffers from AIDS because her mother was infected. She was born two months premature, and there has rarely been a time when she has not been sick. Her entire life has been spent in a public hospital, much of it in intensive care. Placement in a foster care setting was successful, but Debra will need frequent rehospitalization. The institution hopes that Debra will soon be well enough to live with her foster parents, but the staff knows that she will be back.

Hospital costs for treating Debra have been very high, especially since her condition has required many days in intensive care and specialty services. Medicaid has paid for much of the bill. Still, the hospital's public sector revenues have not met all costs.

Cases such as these are typical of the case load in our public hospitals. AIDS is the current dominant problem, and it is a problem that is not likely to disappear. Unfortunately, AIDS strikes many of the already disenfranchised—drug users and the children born to them—and because of its debilitating effects, it usually depletes the resources of its other victims as they attempt to pay for their hospital and nonhospital treatment. It has become commonplace that "almost everyone who dies of AIDS dies broke." Within this fact lies a corollary: public hospitals have become the primary providers for many AIDS patients who cannot afford to pay for their own care.

This is not the first time our public hospitals have faced problems resulting from devastating epidemics. Cholera, smallpox, and polio epidemics each ravaged the nation and tested the limits of the medical community of their times. For the most part, the home and hospital were the primary treatment centers, with public hospitals quickly taking on the role of repository for the afflicted poor, the incurable, and the socially unacceptable. In each case, when the scourge first appeared, only palliative care could be provided to the patients. Eventually, more successful treatment and cures were found as the health care establishment responded to the crises.

Like these earlier epidemics, AIDS is taking a tragic toll on an increasing number of people across the country. The current epidemic is concentrated in large cities, and so it is the nation's large metropolitan area public hospitals that are poised at the front line of the battle against this dread disease. These hospitals have assumed a disproportionate and growing share of AIDS care in the United States. Today, for a number of these public hospitals located in areas

hit early and hard by the AIDS epidemic, this disproportionate share has already become a crushing burden that
has caused financial distress and disruption of service to
patients with AIDS and to other patients as well. The dra-
matic increase in diagnosed cases across the country, and
the projections for future caseloads, illustrates the alarming fact that many other hospitals may soon find themselves facing similar crises.

Chapter 2
Chronic Problems—
Current Consequences

Historically, our nation's public hospitals have often had to struggle to perform their responsibilities effectively.* Always subject to the political and economic conditions of their localities, many of these institutions have been chronically underfunded. As other facilities have avoided treating unattractive or unprofitable patients, they have provided a disproportionate amount of care to the medically indigent. Since many of their patients have no recourse to other providers, these institutions have been

---

* The term "public hospital" includes more than city- or county-owned institutions. Public hospitals are often operated by hospital districts and authorities, states, or state universities. Some have been reorganized into quasi-governmental hospitals that operate as private institutions. In all, they constitute about a third of the nearly six thousand acute care hospitals in the United States today, numbering 1,600–1,900 institutions. Among our public hospitals are a large minority of urban hospitals, more than half of all rural hospitals, and many university teaching hospitals.[1]

The core of this group is made up of about one hundred publicly owned hospitals and hospital systems in our large cities. Averaging five hundred beds, these are big hospitals, major teaching hospitals, and most of their funds are provided by state and local governments and Medicaid.

forced to serve as primary care providers, as well as specialists and sources of tertiary care. They have also assumed social service and alternate care roles in circumstances in which individuals cannot be discharged to a community or a subacute setting.

For example, nursing home beds are now at a premium in many communities. Moreover, subacute facilities in general prefer not to accept public hospital patients, who they tend to perceive as disruptive and requiring greater care than they usually offer. And some public hospital patients, such as drug users or the homeless, may require supervised residential placement that is simply not available.

In general, the 1980s brought a deterioration of the public hospital situation. A report on hospital care to the poor by the Washington-based Urban Institute found that during 1980, one hundred urban public institutions, which represent 6 percent of the hospital beds nationwide, provided 40 percent of the charity care, 19 percent of the bad-debt care, and 12 percent of the Medicaid care (expressed in dollars) in the United States.[2] Between 1980 and 1982, public hospitals in large cities increased the portion of resources devoted to bad-debt and charity care from 17.8 to 19.8 percent, an increase of 11 percent in two years. This commitment far exceeded that of other hospitals.[3]

Information on city public hospitals indicates that this trend has not abated. In 1986, almost 26 percent of the 167,184 inpatient days at member hospitals was defined as bad-debt/charity care.[4] By 1987, this proportion had increased 8 percent, to 28 percent of 180,062 patient days.[5]

To pay for their services to low-income populations, public hospitals have drawn from three sources, singly or in combination: Medicaid, state governments, and local governments. The National Association of Public Hospitals (NAPH), an organization that represents approximately one hundred large metropolitan area hospitals, reports that its members receive on average an estimated 60 percent of their revenues from these sources. Meanwhile, they are less able to rely on revenues from private insurance payments to cover nonpaying patients, since these payers now represent only 12 percent of their revenues.

It has also become unrealistic to rely on state and local payment sources to support an increasing public sector burden. Many state-wide propositions were enacted in the late 1970s and early 1980s to control the growth of property taxes, which have been a very important source of health care dollars. Adding to the pressures on hospital funding, the federal government has phased out general revenue sharing, whereby states received a sum of money to use for public purposes in any way they chose. The hospitals have also had to compete with efforts to increase support for other programs such as education and transportation. Thus, it is unlikely that public institutions will receive adequate financial relief from public sources.

These funding problems, along with the increased demand for indigent care (of which AIDS is a part), come at a time when public hospitals are facing alarmingly high occupancy rates and intolerable pressures on services. In a December 1988 *New York Times* article, Dr. Lewis Goldfrank, director of emergency medicine at Bellevue Hospital Center, commented that patients "are crowding into our corridors, our waiting rooms and our treatment areas. . . . Over the last six months, most of our [public] hospitals have faced changing census patterns that make bed accessibility for the next patient impossible." The prime causes cited in this profile are "AIDS, drug abuse and poverty-related deterioration in health."[6]

The American Hospital Association has reported that occupancy rates for community hospitals in general have been declining, from 76 percent in 1976 to 66 percent in 1986. For city public hospitals, however, the rates have been considerably higher. In 1984, occupancy rates at these institutions averaged 79 percent, and they have remained above 80 percent since 1986. It is not uncommon to see NAPH member hospitals pressed beyond 100 percent of their capacity.[7]

Who is filling these beds? Certainly, public hospitals have not seen a great surge of well-to-do patients. In fact, trends indicate that the number of uninsured individuals has increased significantly, and Medicaid has not kept pace with insurance needs. In fact, during the 1980s Medicaid coverage of individuals at or below the federal poverty level fell from 64 percent to 40 percent. This disenfranchised population looks to the public hospitals for its health care.

AIDS and the Medically Indigent

The well-established pattern of public hospitals treating the medically disenfranchised has never been more evident than in their care of people with AIDS. Although private hospitals continue to be willing to accept AIDS patients with insurance, those AIDS patients without any kind of insurance, as well as those on Medicaid, must frequently rely on public institutions for their care. Those who have been unable to maintain their insurance payments are also unlikely to find treatment at private institutions; those with policies that are inadequate to cover all their service needs are also finding that their options are limited.

Public hospitals across the country have expressed great concern that they are becoming "de facto" AIDS hospitals. Many of these institutions, which treat low-income people with AIDS in their communities or regions, have come to realize that other hospitals are referring AIDS patients to them. One way in which some hospitals may be deflecting AIDS patients is by avoiding developing sophisticated infectious disease departments or other AIDS-related services, thereby requiring that AIDS patients be referred to facilities that offer these services, often public hospitals.

Another common phenomenon is that AIDS patients who are covered by private insurance are finding that drugs such as zidovudine or aerosolized pentamidine, or services that are not inpatient services, are not covered by their insurance. Public hospitals often provide the only recourse. One public hospital, in profiling its AZT treatment protocols, recently listed as its number one financing issue dealing with privately insured AIDS patients whose AZT treatments are not covered by their insurance.

The result of these and other factors is that the relatively few metropolitan area public hospitals are caring for an enormous proportion of persons with AIDS, while projections point to an escalating burden for the foreseeable future.

In New York City, for example, the Office of Strategic Planning of the Health and Hospitals Corporation issued a report in 1988 entitled "The Crisis Overcrowding in New York City Public Hospitals." The report cited the "changing patterns of illness," noting that patients are staying in hospitals longer and explicitly stating that AIDS is the major cause. The average length of stay of AIDS patients is 23.4 days, in comparison with only 9.7 days for the average medical-surgical patient. Meanwhile, the number of AIDS patients in New York City hospitals nearly doubled between December 1986 and December 1987, going from an average of 233 to 426 at any one point in time.

The continual spread of AIDS, added to the sheer number of patients seeking care in public hospitals, directly affects the operation of these institutions. With many public facilities already stretched to capacity in New York, Los Angeles, Dallas, Miami, and elsewhere, waiting lines continue to lengthen for "nonessential" care. Hospitals known for their excellence in treating AIDS patients, which already bear a sizable burden of care in their communities, are suffering immediate consequences.

For example, San Francisco General accounts for 32 percent of all AIDS hospitalization in its area. It also already treats a large number of low-income patients. Recently, the hospital has been forced to divert some of its patients to other hospitals due to an extremely high occupancy rate. Which patients have been diverted? Most often they are patients with private insurance, since San Francisco General's mission, not necessarily shared by other local facilities, is to provide service to all patients, especially those with no other recourse for care. Obviously, such actions have dire ramifications for San Francisco General's financial stability.

Some Implications

Since persons with AIDS are not the only medically indigent group in America in the 1980s, the nation's public hospitals, especially those located in major metropolitan areas, are caring for the large and growing numbers of patients who have little to sustain them. This is a disturbing and growing phenomenon. It is estimated that at least 37 million Americans lack health insurance, and many more are underinsured. The burden of their care has fallen increasingly upon these hospitals, which have traditionally assumed the role of "safety net institutions."

Reflection on health care for the disadvantaged during the past ten years leaves the impression of a troubled era. It is a time replete with examples of neglect, overburdened public hospital systems—some on the verge of collapse—and an overall, marked deterioration in the nation's health care safety net. The AIDS epidemic has brought these weaknesses and failings into much sharper focus. In many ways it serves as a tragic metaphor for problems faced by other patient populations. Any person who has faced the hardships of obtaining the range and quality of care required for elderly patients, Alzheimer's disease victims, or children and adults needing long-term care has faced the very problems facing a person suffering from AIDS. Society's compassion and attention to the needs of people with AIDS in many ways reflect its attitude toward many other populations in need, now and in the future.

By placing an increasingly greater strain on services and providers, the AIDS epidemic has laid bare what many have chosen to ignore in the past. At the same time, since it will not disappear, AIDS demands a response from the country. Will we do as little as possible? Will we recognize a need to act but only tinker around the edges? Or will we adopt a call to action and develop a compassionate, strong, and comprehensive response?

Those who ask, "Why should I care about AIDS?"—or those who believe it has no relevance, currently or potentially, to them—need look no further than the situation in our metropolitan public hospitals. If the AIDS epidemic is left unaddressed, especially in the context of other health care dilemmas, it may only be a matter of time before its effects are felt by insured and uninsured alike. The community facility known, for example, for its quick and effective emergency services may not be able to respond as well because of the need to divert resources for AIDS care. The public hospital known for providing the finest prenatal intensive care in the city may be unable to maintain the quality that had become its hallmark. The public hospital that serves as a regional referral center on which so many suburban and rural areas are dependent may no longer be able to accept patients. The public hospital that attracted the highest-quality medical school graduates may no longer be viewed as a desirable placement for residents.

These are just a few of the possible consequences that

may be awaiting the public hospitals of our cities and counties in the era of AIDS. In their long and distinguished history, our nation's public hospitals have grown to serve a
variety of critical health care functions. It is important to
remember that these institutions, currently strained to the
breaking point by AIDS and other factors, are a vital national resource.

Chapter 3
Urban Public Hospitals: An Endangered National Resource

The public hospitals are an anomaly. They are public institutions in a health care market that is largely privately owned. More importantly, in treating the unprofitable medically indigent populations, they have assumed a role that, although necessary, no one else wants. Some of these institutions have made medical history, and many have been prestigious training grounds for physicians. Yet many have been badly neglected in recent years.

The Contribution of Urban Public Hospitals

The large city hospitals in the United States are distinguished by the sheer volume of the care they provide, by their major role in educating physicians and other health care workers, and by their many vital and often unprofitable services like burn centers and trauma centers. Their hallmark, of course, is the commitment to serving people without regard for their ability to pay.

Who are the people these hospitals serve? Contrary to popular belief, many of today's medically indigent individuals are workers or their dependents. A full two-thirds of the uninsured, for example, are either full-time workers or their dependents.[1] There are many people who have

15

fallen through the cracks of our health care system in one way or another: underinsured people, those who are catastrophically ill and cannot meet their bills, employees of small businesses, and part-time employees. Among them, too, are unemployed individuals who have no health insurance, poor people who do not qualify for Medicaid, and insured people who are disqualified from treatment because they had "preexisting conditions." Finally, there are "special populations," like drug users, prostitutes, the homeless, and people with AIDS. Many of these people, of course, are seriously ill, and not a few are transferred to public hospitals from private hospitals that will not or cannot treat them. This proliferation of indigent constituents has earned the public hospitals the epithets "national health insurance by default" and "family doctor for the poor."

Metropolitan area public hospitals provide a volume of care that is disproportionate to their number. In 1986, for example, forty-eight urban public hospitals admitted 819,166 inpatients, an average of 19,060 per hospital; in the same urban areas other hospitals averaged only 7,038 admissions each. Public hospitals also dominated the outpatient services arena, with an average of 242,00 visits per hospital, in comparison with 60,414 for other short-term community hospitals. Just one year later, in 1987, that number jumped to 278,000 visits per hospital.

The list of distinguished names who have been associated with public teaching hospitals is a long one, including Benjamin Rush, who taught at Philadelphia General; Christian Fenger of Cook County Hospital; and Andre Cournand and Dickinson Richards, two Nobel Prize winners from Bellevue.[2]

City public hospitals have also maintained their commitment to teaching. In 1986, just forty-two of these hospitals trained 8,800 residents, 12 percent of all the residents that were trained in the United States that year.[3] They averaged 173 residents per hospital in 1986, with a ratio of 0.36 residents per bed. (The Council of Teaching Hospitals considers 0.26 a major teaching commitment.)[4]

Besides providing a large volume of services to the poor and training many of our best physicians and other health care professionals, public hospitals offer some very important specialized services that other hospitals do not have, often because these services are not profitable. For example, they are three times more likely than other hospitals to have trauma centers: 76 percent of the urban public hospitals provide these services, compared to 24 percent of other hospitals.

The public hospitals are much more apt to have designated burn centers, neonatal intensive care units, coronary care units and open-heart surgery, and psychiatric services. They also offer a disproportionate share of organized outpatient services. While only 69 percent of the nonpublic hospitals offer outpatient services, 100 percent of the metropolitan area public hospitals do, which makes them, as was noted above, the de facto family doctor for many who cannot afford to have a doctor at all.

A Brief History

Public hospitals date back to the 1730s, when they were founded as "almshouses," patterned after an English institution that housed an assortment of people who had no families or other sources of support: unwed mothers, orphans, alcoholics, the elderly, the mentally ill, and victims of contagious diseases. By the nineteenth century, physicians and social reformers separated the various populations, for example by sending children to orphan asylums and the mentally ill to mental institutions. Those who remained were the people who needed medical care.

Physicians, volunteers, and others helped upgrade the hospitals, improve conditions in general, and develop them into fine training facilities. Various local politicians, including renowned figures like Mayor James Curley of Boston and Governor Huey Long of Louisiana, became vocal proponents of public hospitals, helping to build them into giant institutions. Cook County Hospital in Illinois was typical, growing from 1,360 beds in 1910 to 3,260 in 1960. In the postwar era, spurred by a 1946 law that made public funds available to construct hospitals, many rural areas also built public hospitals.

A turning point in the history of public hospitals was the 1966 passage of the laws that created Medicaid and Medicare. At that time, many patients began to take advantage of the option of using private hospitals. Urban public hospitals responded by reducing the number of beds sharply. Between 1960 and 1980 the number of public hospital beds shrank 38.3 percent, while those in private hospitals increased by 60.6 percent. Despite some predictions of their demise, the public hospitals did not disappear. In fact, the reverse happened. In many states, Medicaid and Medicare began by paying relatively well for their participants, although coverage generally declined in a short time. Though the situation varied widely from state to state, on average, at its height in 1977, Medicaid sponsored 92 percent of those living below the federal poverty line; by 1986, it covered between 38 and 42 percent.[5]

A well-known 1977 study of public hospitals, the Kellogg Commission Report, found that the occupancy rates in public hospitals were higher than had been expected at that high point in the history of government support. The overall average was 69.9 percent, with university facilities averaging 76.6 percent and urban public hospitals in large cities 73.7 percent. Also, these public hospitals were still training nearly 40 percent of all medical and dental residents and 20 percent of other health care professionals.[6]

The 1980s in Context

The crisis conditions that public hospitals are currently facing may be better understood if they are viewed from a historical perspective. Serious overcrowding has happened in the past. During the 1920s and 1930s, in the wake of the depression and widespread unemployment, public hospitals were chronically overburdened in Baltimore, Chicago, Washington, D.C., and other cities. Then as now, the core of the matter was economic. In the 1930s, there were large numbers of people who were unemployed and could not afford to pay.

Today the problem is somewhat more complex. There are, as has been noted, growing numbers of uninsured and underinsured Americans; the Census Bureau has estimated that they have increased 40 percent since 1980. There is also the cost-consciousness that has been prevalent in the health care industry, as it has in the business world in general. Public funds like Medicaid, which were more plentiful in the prosperous 1960s and 1970s, have tended to shrink in this decade of budget deficits and attempts to cut back on government spending. Many state and local governments have also been chronically short of funds. The situation is much worse in states that have been hard hit by economic troubles. As we shall see, the public hospitals are particularly hard pressed in many of the once rapidly growing Sunbelt areas.[7]

Typically, urban public hospitals have been losing money. Revenues are failing to cover costs, leaving 48 percent of the NAPH member hospitals with deficits in 1987. The average deficit of these hospitals in that year exceeded $16 million.[8]

The Current Crisis

In the wake of these pressures, many public hospitals have had to cut back their services and personnel. Some have even had to close their doors. The Kellogg Commission counted ninety major urban public hospitals in 1977. During the past ten years, seven have closed and another ten have been reorganized as private, nonprofit corporations. The remainder have been fighting an increasingly difficult battle to continue providing health care to our nation's neediest patients.

The current crisis in the public hospitals, outlined in the last chapter, was summarized by Larry S. Gage, president of the National Association of Public Hospitals, in his March 1, 1989, appearance before the House Ways and Means Committee:

> In Chicago, Los Angeles, Kansas City, New Orleans, and many other cities the story is the same: Trauma centers and emergency rooms are overcrowded to the breaking point. Occupancy rates continue to rise, topping 100 percent in some cities, and critically ill patients wait up to 36 hours for an inpatient bed. Drug abuse, gang violence, AIDS, the homeless, refugees, and other problems new in the 1980s are growing at an alarming rate in some cities— greatly compromising and in some cases even crowding out their ability to serve less seriously ill indigent patients. . . . [M]any hard-pressed state and local governments are struggling simply to maintain their current level of support, or are actually reducing that support.[9]

It is no longer unusual to hear about public hospitals' inability to obtain resources adequate to meet the needs of their patients:

The situation in Louisiana. In 1987, Lousiana's unemployment rate was 12 percent, double the national average.

The nation's second poorest state, Louisiana had 18.6 percent of its population already living below the federal poverty level at the time of the last census, compared with 12.4 percent nationwide.

Louisiana has the lowest average life expectancy in the nation, very high infant mortality rates, a high percentage of births to teenage mothers, and a high incidence of low-birth-weight babies. The income requirement for a Louisiana household to receive Medicaid is 23.6 percent of the federal poverty level; this means that a family with an income of only 24 percent of the federal poverty level has too high a financial base to receive Medicaid in the state. With more than 800,000 people living in poverty, Louisiana had only 432,807 Medicaid recipients in 1988.

The enormous impact of its economic crisis has aggravated the problems already existing as the result of a historically restrictive Medicaid program for the poor. As a result, the Charity Hospital system has been among the victims of its budget reductions. Even as the demand for services to its medically indigent population rises continuously, the state has had to cut its budget allocations year after year. In 1986, the Charity Hospital system received more than $242.6 million. By 1989, that amount had been cut to about $187.3 million.

To meet these severe restrictions, the hospital system was forced to cut back 244 beds and to close entire units, ranging from inpatient cardiac catheter labs to urology clinics, dermatology clinics, diabetes education, mammography services, and weekend walk-in clinics. Many other services were severely reduced.[10]

The situation in New York City. A recent series of articles in *Newsday* described New York's public hospitals as "struggling to stay afloat in a roiling sea of problems," numbering among them "jammed wards and emergency rooms, uncertain ambulance service, sinking employee morale, and erratic medical treatment."[11] In a 1989 report, State Comptroller Edward Regan concluded that the system was "on the brink of collapse."[12] Employee turnover is very high and the shortage of nurses so acute that it is not unusual to have two registered nurses caring for four wards of forty patients each.

A major cause of the particularly acute situation in New York is the fact that the state, anticipating lower demand, reduced the number of beds by 20 percent in the past eight years. However, the average length of stay began to climb in 1986 and has risen to 9.4 days in 1987 and 10.1 days in 1988. Hospital officials believe that this unexpected change was caused by the AIDS epidemic and the crack epidemic, together with a lack of long-term-care facilities. Occupancy rates are swelling to the breaking point. The occupancy rate for medical-surgical beds increased from 79 percent in 1986 to 98.6 percent in late 1988. It is not uncommon to have severe backups in emergency rooms, because seriously ill people are waiting up to two days for an inpatient bed to become available.

As if these problems were not enough, there is also a looming financial threat. A new reimbursement system in 1988 imperils the hospitals' revenue base: private insurers and Medicaid now pay a fixed rate no matter how long the patient is hospitalized. This is a serious problem for New York City's hospitals, especially in combination with longer stays and bed and staff shortages.[13]

Chapter 4
Profile of the AIDS Crisis

AIDS is national and international in scope, and as is the nature of all epidemics, it is spreading fast. As recently as the summer of 1985, only 12,932 cases of AIDS had been reported to the Centers for Disease Control (CDC). In less than three and a half years, that number had increased almost sevenfold. As of December 26, 1988, some 82,406 individuals had been diagnosed as AIDS victims in the United States.[1] During 1989, the total number of AIDS diagnoses has exceeded 100,000, and recent national estimates project 450,000 cases by 1993.

While our nation leads the world in the number of identified cases, we are not alone. One hundred seventy-seven countries reported 129,385 cases of AIDS by November of 1988.[2] The World Health Organization projects that 10 million people may currently be infected worldwide and that 100 million may be infected by the year 2000.[3] Some experts claim that parts of the African continent have already been devastated by the disease and that Latin America may be following a similar pattern.[4] These estimates indicate that the disease will spread at an exponential pace in the foreseeable future.

New evidence provides alarming projections for carriers of the virus as well. Scientists in San Francisco, reviewing information from a cohort of homosexual men, have concluded that the average incubation period before an infected individual is diagnosed with AIDS is almost eight years, and the upper limit is fifteen years or more. They project that almost all those who are infected with the virus will develop the disease if they do not die from unrelated or other related causes.

At first, AIDS was thought to be primarily a disease of homosexuals; however, major increases in the number of cases in other populations have caused scientists and other experts to change that assumption. During 1985, homosexuals represented 65 percent of the individuals with AIDS in the United States. By the end of 1988, the proportion had declined to 57 percent. For the same period, the number of infected intravenous (IV) drug users increased from 17 to 24 percent. Although children continue to represent a relatively small proportion of the overall estimates, their numbers have increased at an alarming rate as well, from 182 cases in 1985 to 1,298 in 1988.

The spread of AIDS, of course, has resulted in major increases in the health care resources devoted to its treatment. Medium-range estimates placed the per year direct medical care costs at $630 million in 1985, $1.1 billion in 1986, and a projected $8.5 billion by 1991[5] In the mid-1980s, the cost of AIDS health care, while considerable, was less than the health care costs arising from such causes as motor vehicle accidents ($5.6 billion), cancer of the digestive system ($3.0 billion), lung cancer ($2.7 billion), and end-stage renal disease and breast cancer ($2.2 billion each)[6] By 1991, however, only the health-care costs of motor vehicle accidents are projected to be higher than those of AIDS. Hospital care of AIDS patients is expected to utilize 5.9 million inpatient days.

The AIDS Populations in Public Hospitals

Although AIDS sufferers come from all social and economic strata, a large segment either are or become outcasts from the mainstream of health care. As a result, they are likely to encounter great difficulty in receiving the services they require, and because of this, they are likely to be treated at public hospitals (see Tables 1 through 3). Which are the most vulnerable populations? They include the following groups:

- *The working uninsured diagnosed with AIDS.* Many people find that the crippling effects of the disease do not enable them to fulfill their job requirements.
- *People who have exhausted personal resources and/or health insurance benefits.* The current health care system forces AIDS patients and others afflicted with long-term illnesses to "spend down" into poverty. Many Americans are not able to afford either the higher insurance premiums required for high-risk populations or the disproportionate increases in their rates due to their current state of health.
- *IV drug users.* Most of these individuals have no recourse to mainstream health care. In addition, "crack" users who have AIDS frequently spread the disease by prostituting themselves to support their drug habit.
- *Infants and children of mothers who have AIDS.* Large numbers of infants with AIDS are abandoned in the hospitals, often because their mothers have died (boarder babies). Older pediatric patients also typically need continuing care.
- *Dependents who were infected by transfusions.* These include hemophiliac children and low-income elderly whose families can no longer support their care.
- *Victims of sexual abuse.* Some AIDS patients become infected through incest or violent crime and are without sufficient resources to obtain care.
- *The homeless and mentally ill.* These groups frequently are abandoned by the health care system.
- *Minority groups.* Low-income individuals from various

racial and ethnic groups, especially blacks and Hispanics, have been hard hit by the epidemic.

Because of the nature of AIDS, many of the people most at risk (IV drug users and their children and sexual partners) are individuals who would be most likely to seek care at a public institution.

AIDS also strikes otherwise healthy young men, a group who had previously been one of the healthiest and one of the least likely to require any kind of hospital care. According to the Centers for Disease Control, 61 percent of the 82,406 people diagnosed through the end of 1988 as having AIDS were homosexual, and 20 percent were IV drug users. An additional 7 percent were both homosexual/bisexual and drug users. The remaining people with AIDS were either heterosexual (4 percent), blood-product associated (4 percent), children of risk-group members (1 percent), or undetermined (3 percent).[7]

These demographics, however, are changing. The CDC reports that there has been a decrease in the proportion of homosexual cases reported, and an increase in the proportion of IV drug users and heterosexually transmitted cases. In 1988, about 23 percent of the AIDS cases reported were IV drug users, and 5 percent were sexual partners of risk-group members, primarily the sexual partners of drug users. Thus, the biggest growth in AIDS transmission is in the drug-user population. This is a group that is frequently treated at public hospitals, and its growth means a further increase in the percentage of persons with AIDS who will need treatment from public hospitals.

It is not surprising, then, that AIDS patients who are treated in public hospitals differ markedly from those who are treated in other hospitals. Drug use was a factor in the majority (62 percent) of AIDS cases in the National Association of Public Hospital's member hospitals in 1987. Of these, 44 percent were heterosexual drug users, 7 per-

Table 1
Utilization of Services by AIDS Patients
in Public Hospitals

	1985	1987	Percent Change
Hospitals	49	55	12
Patients			
Total	2,977	6,091	105
Average per hospital	61	111	82
Admissions			
Total	4,267	9,116	114
Average per hospital	87	166	91
Inpatient days			
Total	91,091	166,035	82
Average per hospital	1,859	3,019	62
Average length of stay (in days)	21.3	18.2	– 15
Average number of days per patient per year	30.6	27.2	– 11
Average number of admissions per patient per year	1.4	1.5	7

Source: Surveys by the National Association of Public Hospitals, 1985 and 1987 (see Appendix).

Table 2
Demographics: AIDS Patients in Public Hospitals

	Percent 1985*	Percent 1987**	Percent Change
Patient Groups			
Homosexual	41	36	– 5
Homosexual/drug user	5	7	2
Heterosexual/drug user	44	43	– 1
Sex partner of			
risk-group member	4	3	– 1
Child of risk-group member	5	8	3
Blood product	2	2	0
Age			
0–2	5	5	0
3–19	1	2	1
20–49	91	88	– 3
50+	4	6	2
Sex			
Male	84	82	– 2
Female	16	19	3
Race			
Caucasian	23	32	9
Black	45	45	0
Hispanic	28	22	– 6
Other	4	1	– 3

Source: National Public Health and Hospital Institute Surveys, 1985 and 1987.
* Based on 42 hospitals and 2,751 patients.
** Based on 49 hospitals and 5,265 patients.

Table 3
Costs, Charges, and Revenue
(For AIDS Patients and All Patients in Public Hospitals)

	1985*	1987**	Percent Change
Inpatient costs			
Per day	$ 619	$ 649	5%
Per admission	13,185	11,812	– 10
Per patient/year	18,941	17,653	– 7
Inpatient charges			
Per day	761	780	2
Per admission	16,209	14,196	– 12
Per patient/year	23,287	21,216	–9
Inpatient revenues			
Per day	316	361	14
Per admission	6,731	6,570	– 2
Per patient/year	9,670	9,819	2
Inpatient losses (Cost–revenue)			
Per day	303	288	– 5
Per admission	6,454	5,242	– 19
Per patient/year	9,272	7,834	– 16
Other medical/surgical patients			
Cost per day	619	648	5
Charge per day	781	808	3
Revenue per day	486	495	2
Loss per day	133	153	15

Source: Surveys by the National Association of Public Hospitals, 1985 and 1987 (see Appendix).
*Based upon 20 hospitals and 1,866 admissions.
**Based upon 22 hospitals and 2,170 admissions.

cent homosexual drug users, 8 percent children of risk-group members, and 3 percent were sexual partners of risk-group members. Most of the remaining 38 percent of the patients treated were homosexual (36 percent) or people who contracted AIDS from transfusions.

There were also marked differences in the breakdown of the AIDS populations according to sex, race, and age. The CDC reported that 58 percent of all the cases report-ed cumulatively through the end of 1988 were white; the NAPH surveys revealed that 68 percent of the AIDS popu-lation in the public hospitals were nonwhite. While men comprised 91 percent of all AIDS cases, 19 percent of the people with AIDS in public hospitals were female. The public hospitals also treated a disproportionate percentage of children. While only 1 percent of the cases reported to the CDC were two years old or younger, this group made up 5 percent of the AIDS cases in the public hospitals.[8]

Patterns of Medical Care

The types of patients treated in public hospitals present special problems in treatment and in financing. IV drug users are frequently in poor health overall prior to contract-ing AIDS; this prolongs and complicates their treatment. Drug users have been reported to stay in the hospital sig-nificantly longer than other people with AIDS.[9] In addi-tion, drug users frequently have very unstable living situations, may have no support system at home, or may in fact have no home, making discharge planning difficult and often requiring that they stay in the hospital long be-yond the time period that is medically necessary. Treat-ment of children with AIDS, especially children born to AIDS-infected mothers, is especially difficult. These chil-dren are born into unstable families that have very little ability to care for a sick child at home. Often there is no father, and the mother is too ill to care for the child. These children are sometimes abandoned at the hospital, leaving health care workers with the task of finding foster care settings for infants with AIDS.

In most areas of the country, the locus of care for such AIDS patients remains the inpatient hospital unit. Although there are some programs that provide more appropriate care in a more humane and cost-effective way, financing patterns still favor inpatient services.

In 1985, NAPH member hospitals treated an average of 61 people with AIDS as inpatients, averaging 87 admissions and 1,859 days. By 1987, the number of patients treated had increased 82 percent, to 111 persons with AIDS per facility, 166 admissions and 3,019 inpatient days. By contrast, the average private hospital treated only 36 persons with AIDS in 1987.[10]

As caseloads increase in hospitals with already high occupancy rates, the hospitals will need to look for ways of decreasing lengths of stay where appropriate. For example, as hospitals gain experience in treating AIDS, it may be possible for outpatient programs to replace some inpatient services. Learning from experience, NAPH facilities reported decreases in average lengths of stay, from 21.3 days in 1985 to 18.2 days in 1987, while the average number of admissions per patient per year increased slightly, from 1.4 to 1.5. The total number of days patients spent in the hospital was down slightly between 1985 and 1987, from 30.6 to 27.2. However, average lengths of stay were highest in the Northeast, where hospitals treated more IV drug users.

Most hospitals provide care to AIDS patients throughout the hospital, placing each patient on a ward most appropriate for his or her needs. In contrast, six of fifty public hospitals had established units dedicated solely to AIDS patients by the end of 1987. The hospitals that have established such units tend to be those with very large caseloads. They average more patients in-house than there are beds on the

AIDS unit, and use the units for evaluation, referring many of the patients out to other hospital units.

AIDS patients are most likely to be treated in an acute care unit. Of inpatient days, 89 percent were recorded as general acute care services, 3 percent as intensive care, and 8 percent as "medically ready for discharge," a situation in which the patient is medically cleared to leave but no appropriate discharge placement has been found. In the Northeast, 11 percent of all days were spent waiting for appropriate discharge. These patients may be waiting for skilled nursing care, hospice service, foster care, or other institutional care that is either scarce or unavailable to patients without insurance to cover the costs. Others have chaotic home situations that preclude their returning home, and still others have no home to return to. These "medically ready for discharge" days present vexing problems for a public hospital that has an overflowing census and other patients waiting for service.

In addition to their inpatient services, public hospitals also provide a great deal of service to AIDS patients on an outpatient basis, and the volume of this care is increasing rapidly. In 1985, NAPH member hospitals provided an average of 965 outpatient visits per facility. By 1987, these hospitals were averaging 1,539 visits per facility. Individual patients averaged seven outpatient visits per year in 1985 and nine visits per year in 1987.

As caseloads increase, more hospitals will find it useful or perhaps necessary to track outpatient service use so they can coordinate their AIDS care more efficiently. Public hospitals have already begun feeling the pressure to manage their care to AIDS patients because of the volume of care they provide and because so much of it is unsponsored. By 1987, 46 percent of the NAPH member hospitals had implemented some type of case management program for AIDS patients, especially in the Northeast, where 79 percent of the public hospitals had a case management system.

Many hospitals, particularly public hospitals, have also taken the lead not just in treatment of AIDS but in prevention and education programs. To this end, many hospitals have found it valuable to link up with groups in the community that represent individuals at high risk for AIDS. These groups can assist the hospitals in reaching the high-risk populations. By 1987, 73 percent of metropolitan public hospitals had established ties with groups representing the gay community, and 60 percent had formed links with groups representing IV drug users; 64 percent had formed ties with minority groups, and 52 percent with groups of women at risk.

Financing

The bill for AIDS is high. The average urban public hospital spent almost $2 million on AIDS inpatient care in 1987 and $244,700 on outpatient care. The average hospital lost almost $900,000 on inpatient services and almost $200,000 on outpatient services. These losses represent a very wide range, from a low of $3,656 to a high of $3,143,364. For the twenty-two hospitals that reported information on the cost of AIDS care, losses totaled more than $23 million.

Government support has been the financial lifeblood of public institutional care to people with AIDS. However, the disease is presenting an exceedingly difficult dilemma. It has placed an additional financial burden squarely on public hospitals and their resources at a time when indigent care has been perceived as a major national problem. The inability of some communities to shoulder the increased financial burden has required the rationing of care to AIDS patients, along with other indigent populations.

During 1987, in one southwestern public hospital that receives only 30 to 40 percent of its support from public and private third-party payers, indigent patients who were qualified to receive AZT treatment were told that the institution could not cover the costs of their care. The draconian result in this situation was that the primary provider of care to those who could not afford to pay turned these individuals away. Other chief executive officers of public facilities have voiced the still unanswered question: "How am I going to pay for the care these AIDS patients need?"

Even in cities where the inpatient reimbursement is adequate, the hospital may lose millions of dollars on unnecessary inpatient care, because it cannot find suitable outplacements. This situation demonstrates another major financing problem: lack of coverage for nonhospital AIDS services. Current financing strategies for alternative care fall far short for two primary reasons: reimbursement is not enough to stimulate providers to develop or expand nonhospital services for AIDS patients, and the mechanisms for setting up these services either do not exist or are hampered by complex requirements.[11] For example, effective home- and community-based care frequently cannot be accomplished without additional financial support. Medicaid allows states the option of applying for waivers to establish such care for AIDS patients; however, Medicaid requires a proposal to assure that a program will need no additional expenditures beyond the current levels for the targeted patient populations.

State and local governments, also concerned with the rising costs of care to low-income populations, often fear that support for additional services will "open the financing floodgates," resulting in an exponential increase in costs. Thus, these entities have also tended to fund only the most pressing services or, at best, to keep any innovative efforts small and local.

The financial story is a grim one. The costs of AIDS are high, the revenues do not meet the costs, and the sources of funds are drying up.

Inpatient care. In 1985, the average cost per diem of caring for an AIDS patient in a metropolitan public hospital was $619. Since the average length of stay was 21.3 days, the cost per admission averaged $13,185. In the course of a year, the average patient incurred $18,941 in inpatient expenses. Revenues met only 51 percent of the costs, so that the hospitals lost an average of about $300 per day, more than $6,000 on each admission and $9,000 on each patient during the year. The costs per day for AIDS patients were identical to the costs of treating other medical-surgical patients, but revenues were considerably higher for other medical-surgical patients, at $486 per day, as compared with slightly more than $300 per day for AIDS patients.

By far the largest source of payment for AIDS care in public hospitals is Medicaid. In 1985, 62 percent of the AIDS admissions to public hospitals were paid by Medicaid; by 1987, that fell to 54 percent. The next-largest category of payment is "self-pay and other," representing almost exclusively patients with no source of insurance, cases for which the hospital will get no reimbursement. Frequently called "no-pay," this category constituted one-fourth of all admissions to metropolitan public hospitals in 1985 and one-third of all admissions in 1987.

For public hospitals, only 9 percent of all 1987 AIDS admissions were covered by private insurance, up very slightly from 8 percent in 1985. The remaining admissions were covered by some sort of public funding, either Medicaid, Medicare, prisoner funds, or the public hospital budget allocation from the local government. (However, not every public hospital receives funds from the local government that operates it.) The sources of financing in a public hospital differ a great deal from those in the typical private hospital, which gets almost half its payments for AIDS care from private insurance. For private hospitals, only 13 percent of admissions fall into the "self-pay" category.[12]

Because Medicaid is a program that is administered by the states, the levels of coverage and the proportion of the poor population that is covered differ widely. In many southern states, Medicaid covers a very small portion of the population below the poverty line. According to Health Care Financing Administration Program statistics, the Medicaid programs in Florida, Texas, Alabama, Arkansas, Tennessee, Virginia, South Carolina, Georgia, and Louisiana all cover less than 31 percent of the population below the federal poverty line. Of the southern states, only the District of Columbia and Maryland are above the national average, and they cover only about half of those below the federal poverty line. The remaining poor population has virtually no health care coverage, relying on the public hospital to provide free care.[13] The situation in the South illustrates the importance of the Medicaid program to the financing of AIDS care. In 1987, only 18 percent of the public hospital AIDS patient population was covered by Medicaid, and 68 percent had neither public not private insurance. Public hospitals in the South lost over $8,000 per patient per year, more than any other region—demonstrating that states' Medicaid policies have a direct effect on hospitals' AIDS revenues, and perhaps also on patients' access to health care.

Outpatient care. In 1987, urban public hospitals reported an average cost per visit for AIDS patients of $159, and an average cost per patient per year for outpatient services of $1,749. Revenues covered only 26 percent of the costs, an average of $41 per visit, and losses averaged almost $1,300 per patient per year. In contrast, the costs for non-AIDS outpatient visits averaged only $105, and revenues were higher at $51. Thus, the loss per visit was half that of the AIDS patients.

It has been difficult to collect information about sources of payment for outpatient services, because of difficulties in tracking the use of these services by people with AIDS. In 1987, out of a reported 7,543 visits, 64 percent were self-pay visits, 24 percent were covered by Medicaid, 10 percent were covered by private insurance, and the remaining 2 percent were Medicare visits. The alarmingly high proportion of self-pay or no-pay visits points to a significant problem for public hospitals. Clearly, there is currently no financial incentive for these institutions to provide more outpatient care, even if such care is more cost-effective and more appropriate for the patient.

Emerging Problems for Public Hospitals

The AIDS crisis poses some formidable, yet familiar, problems for public hospitals, along with issues that, either by nature or by degree, they have not previously encountered.

Staffing. Doctors and nurses enter their professions believing that they will be able to help their patients. While they realize that some of their patients will not recover, personal morale is dependent in part on improving patients' condition and quality of life.

AIDS has starkly altered these expected outcomes. The professionals who minister to afflicted infants, children, and adults frequently perform only a palliative function. They find themselves capable of only temporarily staving off inevitable decline and encounter death with virtually every individual they see. Frequently, even their ability to ease pain and suffering is limited. Eventually, the stresses of caring for this population and the inability to change the course of this tragic disease, especially for the young, take their toll on medical professionals. The result is "burnout," medical professionals who are emotionally and psychologically spent.

Public hospitals have worked to train and educate their staffs about this phenomenon. They have altered work patterns and shifted staff where possible. But burnout remains a serious problem for everyone who is coping with the AIDS epidemic.

Public hospitals treating large numbers of AIDS patients also suspect that there is a growing reluctance among many graduating medical students to train at their institutions. In addition, some of these institutions have reported concern that the AIDS epidemic is affecting their ability to recruit the high-caliber medical staff they have historically relied on to meet their patient care needs. For medical school graduates, the hallmark of public hospital training has been exposure to a full spectrum of medical care experiences. This expectation is compromised by the urgent need to render AIDS care. The result is that public hospitals are unable to fill their medical staff positions with the high-quality students they have traditionally been able to attract.

Treating a new and more seriously ill population. Many AIDS patients at public hospitals would traditionally receive health care at these institutions. However, this epidemic has disproportionately infected a younger population, consisting of many individuals who would not normally have needed care at all, let alone at the level required by AIDS. The emergence of this new patient population has major consequences for the public hospitals. Since the great majority of these patients are likely to be poor, financial support must be obtained from an already stretched public sector. Indeed, for all the levels of government that support AIDS care, the incapacitation of a population that customarily contributes taxes has had serious financial ramifications.

Nor are public health systems prepared to cope with some new patient populations that have additional health care needs. For example, Jackson Memorial Hospital in Miami has experienced an increase in newborn AIDS patients. Many of these infected babies are Haitians who were abandoned at the hospital while their infected mothers returned to their homeland and died. These Jackson Memorial children, whose care is very expensive, are not easily placed in foster homes and need continual care and treatment.

Another emerging population that is causing increasing concern for public hospitals is that of human immunodeficiency virus (HIV)-infected individuals who have not been diagnosed with AIDS but are nonetheless very ill. Early studies in New York City have documented higher than expected numbers of IV-drug-using patients who are HIV-infected and are succumbing to illnesses related to their compromised immune systems. If the consequences of HIV infection experienced in New York City are borne out nationwide in the future, the health care system will face yet another exponential increase in demands for care.

The rise in inner-city use of "crack" cocaine has also created a new HIV-infected population. As New York City's health commissioner, Stephen Joseph, recently stated, "Crack and the hypersexuality associated with it—including sex-for-drugs transactions—have led to increases in genital ulcer disease, HIV transmission and HIV infection."[14] Once again, inner-city public hospitals will bear the brunt of providing care for the complex medical needs of these individuals.

In many cities, too, the public hospitals are realizing that the AIDS patients they treat are more severely ill than AIDS patients in general. Recent studies of the AIDS population treated in New York City have demonstrated that the public hospital patients—including disproportionate numbers of IV drug users and children—are, indeed sicker than those treated in private hospitals.[15] The public institutions themselves have to find a way to pay the bill for the additional resources that are required to meet these patients' health care needs.

Additional institutional costs. Hospitals have generally attempted to document the direct costs of inpatient care to AIDS patients so that they could obtain adequate reimbursement for the most expensive component of treatment. However, institutions that are treating disproportionately large numbers of AIDS patients are incurring additional costs that are not immediately recognized in hospital reimbursement. One relatively new expense that has become common in these hospitals is that of educating and training health care workers about AIDS. Infectious waste disposal has become much more sophisticated with the onset of this epidemic. The increased demand for blood and blood products also has added to the overall hospital costs.

Public hospitals have provided AIDS testing to individuals, and, in Illinois and other states where premarital testing has been required, institutions like Cook County Hospital have been inundated with requests for testing. Another cost has arisen from concerns about discrimination, which have required public hospitals to increase their efforts to preserve confidentiality. The costs of simple supplies such as gloves have risen exponentially, and shortages of these items have required some hospitals to pay a premium to assure an adequate supply.

Public hospitals have had to increase the number of social workers, counselors, mental health staff educators, administrative personnel, screening staff, and others to ensure that staff are sensitive to racial and ethnic issues. Public and private payers often do not recognize the full costs for these essential professionals as additional inpatient expenses.

The needs of HIV-infected patients. During the early years of the AIDS epidemic, diagnosis occurred only after a patient became ill. Many patients died shortly after the acute onset of AIDS-related opportunistic infections. Others lived longer, usually succumbing within two years. Throughout this early period, the medical community could do little to delay the progress of the disease.

Now, although the condition to date has remained almost universally fatal, AZT and other therapies are extending the lives of AIDS patients significantly. Even so, while some individuals will be able to continue to work, many of them will have to rely on personal resources as their illness progresses. In all likelihood, most will eventually come to depend on the public sector for financial, health, and social service assistance. In many areas of the country, this shift from independence to dependence on the public sector has important implications for public hospitals. As these patients live longer, exhaust their resources, become unable to work, and lose their insurance coverage, the public hospitals are likely to bear a disproportionate share of their burden.

Recent AIDS research documents the disease's very long gestation period and emphasizes testing. These developments have created new demands on public hospitals and other health care providers. Many individuals who test positive for the virus are realizing that they should receive treatment for HIV infection even though they do not yet have AIDS. Currently, response to early identification of infection has focused on life-style changes; preventive and experimental use of drugs, especially AZT; monitoring health care status; and treating illnesses before they further weaken the immune system.

The implications of these new developments are unclear

at this time. If the medical community intensifies its efforts to bring HIV-infected individuals into the health care system, providers will be required to devote more resources to early intervention. Moreover, since the period of infection before the onset of AIDS may well average ten years or longer, public hospitals will need to make long-term commitments to these patients.

Efforts of private insurers to limit their liability. Private insurers have been closely monitoring the impact of the AIDS epidemic on their expenditures. While assessments to date have indicated a minimal effect, private insurers are concerned about future trends, what the trends will mean for their policyholder rates, and ultimately, how AIDS will affect their competitiveness. Some consultant groups, such as Claritas Corporation, have taken advantage of this concern. They are marketing profiles of *all* zip codes in the United States.[16] These profiles use census data, CDC data, and HIV infection rates, and other information to determine the risk of writing a health or life insurance policy to individuals who may be HIV-infected. Claritas has attempted to "validate" its profiles by matching its information with magazine subscriptions to homosexually oriented publications.

As they study the situation, insurance companies are beginning to press efforts to require testing. For example, many single males in San Francisco have had difficulty obtaining an individual health insurance policy without submitting to an HIV test. While disenrolling people with AIDS from their policies is illegal, some insurance companies are effectively doing just that by greatly increasing the policy fees of these individuals. For patients who are unable to work, such additional costs become prohibitive, causing some to drop their coverage. These patients then come to depend on public sector support for their care.

The costs and availability of new treatments. The drug AZT is one example of a relatively new and expensive AIDS treatment. When it first became available, AZT therapy averaged nearly $10,000 per year, a level so prohibitive for low-income patients and many of their providers that Congress enacted a law to provide temporary financial assistance to states and localities for the drug. Innovative therapies will become available in the future, but Congress cannot be expected to provide supplemental payment for each of them. Who will pay for these treatments? This critical question must be addressed effectively for both patients and providers if we are to avoid a second question: Who will be excluded?

Chapter 5
Underlying Issues: A National Health Care System in Trouble

AIDS has captured the headlines and the attention of many sectors of American society. As this epidemic touches the lives of more and more citizens, more people will join the debate about what should be done.

One of the major issues that our society must resolve is the type and the intensity of the response it is willing to support. The adequacy of our response to this epidemic may also determine whether many of our nation's public hospitals will continue to fulfill their mission effectively or whether they will become increasingly debilitated by the burden of AIDS care.

While the disease is relatively new, the health-care-related needs of AIDS patients resemble those of other populations requiring comprehensive care. Individuals who are afflicted with AIDS face a health care system and a society that, to date, have not addressed their extensive health care needs. In fact, when one examines closely the shortcomings of health care delivery and treatment for AIDS sufferers and many other patients, an unsettling, familiar pattern of fragmentation and neglect emerges.

In essence, the AIDS epidemic has exposed many of the serious, fundamental problems in our national approach to health care, especially for the disenfranchised. The problems encompass at least three major areas of health care policy: a pattern of neglecting the most vulnerable populations, inconsistent and inadequate financing, and failure to deliver many essential services. The policy issues that affect AIDS patients treated in public hospitals parallel the issues that are raised by the health care situation of low-income populations across the United States. These issues are also closely bound up with the fate of our deeply troubled metropolitan area public hospitals.

A Pattern of Neglecting the Most Vulnerable Populations

What is the country's reaction to the medically disenfranchised? Unfortunately, the United States has a long and disturbing history of neglecting such populations as the chronically mentally ill, the chronically ill, and the poor.

The chronically mentally ill. Nineteenth century America believed that the chronically mentally ill, by the deeds of their lives or by their character, had brought their affliction upon themselves. Somehow, many believed, if these people had led more virtuous lives, they would not have become so ill. As a result of this attitude, the preferred treatment for the chronically mentally ill, at times in our history, was to isolate them.

While current attitudes toward mental illness are more enlightened than those of earlier times, many of the needs of those afflicted remain unmet. Efforts in the 1960s and 1970s to provide more appropriate, community-based care were thwarted by reluctance to expend more resources. The lack of community-based care made inevitable the failure of the deinstitutionalization movement of the past thirty years. Calls for reinstitutionalization have gained strength, especially because of the visible and disturbing phenomenon of the mentally ill homeless on the streets. However, while society struggles with this problem, deinstitution-alization, combined with the inability or unwillingness of other providers to render care, has, by default, placed the responsibility for this population at the doorstep of many inner-city public hospitals.

The chronically ill. Chronically ill patients must cope with a health care system that has never planned effective-ly for their long-term needs. These patients, who require extended medical intervention for a specific condition, fre-quently have difficulty obtaining other health-related sup-port. Individuals suffering from such conditions as multi-ple sclerosis and muscular dystrophy find that little coor-dination of care is available. Moreover, their access to vi-tal care is often overshadowed by the specter of mounting costs. Many cancer patients face extended periods of remis-sion, but are never rid of their affliction and live with the distinct possibility that they will require periodic, costly care. Many of these individuals exhaust their resources and come to receive services only through public sector support.

The poor. The poor also face formidable limitations in access to health services. Historically, people who could not afford to pay for their care were reduced to relying on charity providers, especially public hospitals. In the 1960s, the advent of Medicare and Medicaid expanded the health care options for these individuals, even though inequities remained. In the current competitive environment, how-ever, bottom-line-conscious health care providers tend to concentrate on treating patients who can pay their way with insurance coverage—for the most part, private insur-ance. Frequently, this preference excludes or severely con-strains treatment for the millions of U.S. citizens who lack any kind of health insurance. Health care providers also must place substantial limitations on their acceptance of Medicaid patients, since this payer for low-income health care, in many circumstances, pays less than the provider's costs.

The emphasis on revenue-generating care among health care providers leaves public hospitals and a relatively few private institutions with the responsibility for treating the medically disenfranchised. As a result, the indigent are likely to have great difficulty gaining access to care and receiving the range of services they require.

People with AIDS. AIDS sufferers have much in common with these and other disenfranchised groups. Like the chronically mentally ill of the nineteenth century, they have been shunned by many of their fellow citizens. Ideas for handling the problem have even included transporting New York City AIDS patients to another state, such as West Virginia, where costs would be lower, or to an "abandoned hospital."[1] Many people believe that those with AIDS have brought the condition on themselves and that AIDS is their own fault. The disproportionate number of AIDS patients treated in public hospitals attests to the reluctance of many providers to render care. Like the chronically ill, people with AIDS must plan, as well as they can, for frequent and costly medical care. Their condition will not be cured in the foreseeable future but, at best, will enter a stage of remission. They are likely to use a substantial part of their available resources on long-term care. Like the poor, many will find that their access to services is greatly limited. While they are likely to receive hospital care, other kinds of health care—home- and community-based services in particular—remain grossly inadequate.

Inconsistent and Inadequate Financing

The primary sources of support for the expensive medical needs of people with AIDS are, as noted in Chapter 4, private insurance, Medicaid, and state and local governments. There are, however, significant problems in this system of reimbursement. Most of these problems are common to AIDS and other long-term conditions; many, too, transcend the distinction between public and private sectors. For instance, our payment systems have overemphasized medical care at the expense of health care, thereby discouraging the development of other essential services. In addition, the tendency to use specific categories of funding to encourage certain specific treatments discourages providers from developing a broad spectrum of necessary services.

Medicaid, the primary federal provider of financial support for low-income patients, requires state participation monetarily and administratively. Medicaid coverage varies from state to state, since the federal government allows substantial flexibility in the types of services that states cover and in the categories of eligibility after minimal obligations are met.

In states with liberal Medicaid programs, such as New York and California, public hospitals provide the overwhelming proportion of care to low-income people with AIDS. However, private hospitals in these states also treat a large number of AIDS patients. Generally speaking, private hospitals' acceptance of low-income patients tends to be predicated on their ability to obtain some Medicaid reimbursement for treatment. Even in states with liberal Medicaid programs, many of the public and private hospitals face other financial problems in connection with low-income patients. California, for example, has reduced significantly the level of reimbursement to all health care providers. In a recent statement before the House, California Congressman Pete Stark commented:

> Many [California] hospitals report little or no increases in [Medicaid] payment levels since initial contracts were signed in 1984. Today 10 percent fewer California hospitals accept Medicaid than in 1983. The loser, of course, is the Medicaid beneficiary who cannot gain access to needed hospital services.[2]

Thus, payment to many hospitals, for both inpatient and noninpatient (outpatient and community-based) care, has become "a mile wide and an inch deep."

By far the lowest proportion of care to low-income AIDS patients occurs in the private hospitals in states whose Medicaid programs restrict the optional categories of those who are eligible. For example, the federal government automatically qualifies AIDS patients to receive Social Security Disability Insurance. However, the Medicaid program in Georgia does not allow recipients to apply disability payments to medical care costs in order to reduce their income sufficiently to qualify for Medicaid ("spending down"). Private hospitals in these states can treat far fewer low-income AIDS patients, since they cannot receive any payment whatsoever.

What happens in these situations? States with more restrictive Medicaid programs place even greater pressure on local governments and public hospitals to support AIDS and indigent care. In communities like Dallas, where the state Medicaid program is one of the most restrictive in the nation, the major public hospital for the area, Parkland Memorial Hospital, estimates that 75 percent of the AIDS patients it treats have no insurance coverage, public or private. The annual loss on these patients alone was $3–4 million during 1987–88. Moreover, the cost to Dallas County for bearing the financial burden of the uninsured is substantial: in 1991, the county will expend $57 million to support necessary AIDS care for its residents.

The problems hospitals face in finding financial support for low-income patients are even more acute for non-inpatient care. With few exceptions, Medicaid has offered little incentive for providers to develop more extensive outpatient and community-based programs. Moreover, with state and local governments concentrating on maintaining adequate inpatient services, public hospitals have not found cohesive support for alternatives to the hospital bed.

Failure to Deliver the Range of Essential Services

One of the ongoing, major failures of our health care system is the unavailability of a coordinated, comprehensive continuum of essential services. Nowhere is this situation more apparent than in the case of those with AIDS.

A man or woman with few resources who is diagnosed as AIDS-infected faces many health care obstacles. Very frequently, the acute onset of opportunistic infections requires inpatient treatment. If the hospitalized patient has no support system, as in the case of many AIDS patients treated in public hospitals, it becomes the institution's responsibility not only to provide the necessary acute inpatient care but also to arrange for essential health-related services once that person is discharged from the hospital. If arrangements cannot be made, the hospital becomes the provider of subacute as well as acute care.

What care is required for such a patient? In addition to acute inpatient care, many AIDS patients, especially those treated in public hospitals, may need help in the home, placement in an appropriate nursing or intermediate care facility, sheltered living arrangements, terminal illness assistance, and numerous other services. Even if the low-income patient has an adequate support system, assistance may still be necessary in linking him or her with appropriate services.

Many of the problems AIDS patients have in obtaining access to necessary services are rooted in providers' issues and concerns. A recent report in the *Journal of the American Medical Association* cites studies on house staffs' reluctance to treat AIDS patients and pathologists' refusal to perform autopsies on them.[3] Specific populations, like IV drug users, have encountered rehabilitation programs with long waiting lines. Other essential, community-based services exist only in a planning document and not in reality.

Subacute care facilities present special problems.[4] Aside from the generally known fact that alternative care beds in subacute care facilities are very scarce, many skilled nursing institutions are reluctant to take AIDS patients because the costs of caring for them are believed to be greater than the costs of caring for more typical nursing home patients. Some nursing homes are fearful of the consequences of being perceived as AIDS facilities. Still others are not prepared for the special services required by that patient population.

A Three-Tier System: Threat or Reality?

A debate has been taking place within U.S. health policy circles for many years: Have U.S. health services become a two-tier system? Some argue that this country has one level of care for individuals with private insurance or the wealthy, whose treatment is of incomparable quality and available on demand; by default, a second, inferior level exists for the poor, whose services are rationed and quality of care compromised. The AIDS epidemic has fueled this debate. It also brings up the possibility that a third level might be added, distinct from the other two, for medically indigent individuals who are not eligible for Medicaid.

Hospitals have little problem treating privately insured patients with AIDS or any other illness. This is because reimbursement by private payers generally equals or exceeds costs, and because hospitals have increased their knowledge and sophistication in treating AIDS. These patients are an attractive financial target population. Because hospitals are struggling to survive in a competitive environment, many are offering a level of care and an appealing setting that will bring insured AIDS patients to them. Some private hospitals have even advertised for non-AIDS patients, offering them cash payments for using the inpatient units.

Competition and declining hospital occupancy rates have placed so much pressure on private institutions that many have expanded their acceptable patient universe, focusing on certain Medicaid beneficiaries. While Medicaid is not as generous as private insurance, and varies by state, some well-managed institutions have succeeded in filling beds and receiving reimbursements that are at least sufficient to cover most of their costs. For low-income AIDS patients, such opportunities have afforded some access to high-quality care.

The medically indigent who are not eligible for Medicaid encounter the greatest difficulty in obtaining high-quality care. Since hospital reimbursement for attending to this population is always severely limited, many providers can serve only very small numbers or none at all. Those providers that do accept these patients, such as public hospitals, are frequently filled to capacity and are able to treat only those who need immediate or critical attention.

Many public and private hospitals that serve the medically disenfranchised have claimed that the country, in general, has avoided a tiered system of care. These providers believe that, except for the lack of amenities, treatment in their institutions is no different from that in other institutions. Nevertheless, AIDS and other crises—which result in overworked staffs, facilities stretched beyond their limits, and insufficient resources—are quickly and tragically making more credible the claim that the United States is becoming a multitiered system of care.

In an era dominated by competition and "survival of the fittest institution," there may be little room for AIDS patients and others who are not "profitable." This is the world in which public hospitals attempt to fulfill their mission of serving all, regardless of ability to pay. Nowhere are the pressures of these times more evident than in New York City, where the major providers of health services to low-income and drug-using AIDS patients currently treat 35 percent of this population, although they have only 16 percent of the city's medical/surgical beds. If the situation were left unchanged, by 1991, these institutions would find 25 percent of all their medical-surgical beds filled by people with AIDS.[5]

Chapter 6

The Future of the Nation's Public Hospitals in the Age of AIDS

In 1982, just before AIDS made a significant impact, Harry Dowling wrote a book called *City Hospitals*, in which he dramatically summed up the plight of the public hospitals in a single sentence: "The vital question has always been and still remains: Does anybody care?"[1]

Dowling's question grows more poignant in the context of the AIDS epidemic. Clearly, this illness has left its mark on the nation and its health care system. As the previous chapters have shown, AIDS has placed the greatest strain on a public hospital system that was already overburdened and underfunded. It has also brought considerable public attention to the glaring deficiencies of our current health care system.

How will the nation respond to the intense needs of AIDS patients and other medically disenfranchised Americans? Will we rise to the current challenge? The questions are difficult, dealing with a series of complex issues. As stated in the 1988 report of the Presidential Commission on the Human Immunodeficiency Virus (HIV) Epidemic, some of the central issues are:

- Those who are infected with HIV have "varied and complex" health care needs, which add to the problems of our already overburdened health care system.

55

- The costs of treating people with HIV are very high.
- More and more of these costs are being borne by the public hospitals and such public funding sources as Medicaid and state and local public assistance programs.

The Commission explicitly points out the urgent and far-reaching implications of its findings:

The Commission's examination of health care for persons with HIV-related illnesses has revealed several areas in urgent need of attention which, if given, will not only benefit HIV-infected persons, but will also promote better delivery of care to persons with other chronic illnesses.[2]

The Issues

There is thus clear agreement that, no matter what course of action is taken, this illness has left its mark on the nation and its health care system, and it has provided guidance for the future. By addressing the "urgent needs" of people with AIDS, we will also assist the ranks of similar populations who are medically indigent. In addition to the general health policy issues discussed in Chapter 5, several specific issues must be considered in any attempt to formulate an AIDS policy. The most important of these are the extent of public and private sector involvement with the disease, the role of Medicaid and the federal government, and society's attitudes and prejudices.

The involvement of public and private funding sources. The AIDS epidemic has required public and private providers and supporters of care to question how much responsibility they arc willing to take. Some private insurers believe that the high-risk nature of the disease should allow them to exclude vulnerable populations, even though the cost, spread over all policyholders, is currently minimal. The federal government, to date, has been reluctant to increase its contributions to Medicaid. The states have suggested that Medicaid and other health service contributions are all they can afford. Many overburdened local governments believe that other sectors are not bearing their share of the burden, leaving counties and cities to pick up increasing costs.

Any effort on the part of one sector to abrogate responsibility will virtually guarantee a breakdown of the entire system. It will also be accompanied by recriminations from other funding sources, who will question why they should support AIDS care if a public or private source of support is withdrawn. For instance, a private sector effort to exclude people with AIDS from insurance coverage will call for a proportionate increase in aid from a public sector that is already bearing a disproportionate share. Any attempt by the public sector to make up that loss will become increasingly difficult as the epidemic escalates and the number of indigent AIDS sufferers proliferates.

The role of Medicaid and the federal government. While all payers play essential roles in providing support for AIDS care, Medicaid is the major funding source of the medically disenfranchised. Hospitals, other health care providers, and other payers will be monitoring closely Medicaid's response not only to traditional inpatient and outpatient care but to innovative services as well. Also important are the policies and attitudes of the administration and Congress. They set a tone for the nation. Public responses in the form of support to public hospitals and antidiscrimination hinge in large part on the positions they adopt.

Social attitudes and prejudices. AIDS has left a large segment of our population untouched. While many individuals support continuing research and increasing resources for AIDS patients, a large number are antagonistic or, at best, apathetic to such support. Their reasons vary: they claim that people who have AIDS have brought the illness on themselves through immoral behavior, that AIDS will not affect them in any way, or that other health care problems are more pressing. These and other attitudes are rooted in fear and ignorance. The availability of adequate care will depend on whether or not AIDS is recognized as a societal responsibility and a societal concern. The fact remains that large and growing numbers of people—young and old, male and female, black, white, Hispanic—desperately need care.

Metropolitan area public and private hospitals, many of which are major teaching institutions with excellent reputations, are treating large numbers of AIDS patients. As these facilities are required to devote more resources to AIDS care, it is more likely that other services will be adversely affected, including those that non-AIDS patients may require. Moreover, local governments that devote more resources to combat the epidemic will have to make tough decisions on taxes and on other services such as police, education, roads, and the environment.

The course of our national response will depend heavily on whether we view AIDS in isolation or as an interrelated part of the nation's health care problems. If we believe this illness is distinct and does not affect society as a whole, we will mute the intensity of our response. If we perceive AIDS as an epidemic that presents the same problems that other acute and long-term conditions do, then our response will be more likely to garner widespread support and to have a systemwide effect.

Three Policy Alternatives

The fate of the nation's public hospitals will be guided, if not determined, by the decisions made by supporters and society in general. Moreover, the impact of health care decisions on the AIDS epidemic will determine whether hospitals respond adequately or face a crippling future. The following three possible options for the provision of care are presented along with the potential impact of each on public hospitals and the nation's health care system.

A status quo response. A future in which no change in AIDS financing or services occurs would place the responsibility for care increasingly with the public sector. A larger proportion of AIDS patients will be IV drug users, pediatric cases, and sex partners of current risk groups; this expected shift will increase the number of indigent AIDS patients. Private insurers, seeing their costs increasing and faced with no plan to coordinate support to people with AIDS, would intensify their attempts to reduce coverage. Medicaid would continue to support a large number of AIDS patients, but state-by-state program inequities would accelerate the spread of an uneven national patchwork of AIDS care.

Public hospitals would suffer the most under this scenario. Nationally, there would be no incentives for private providers to treat AIDS patients. In fact, there would be potentially more disincentives, due to higher-cost treatments, more severely ill populations, and poorer patients. Emphasis would remain on inpatient hospital reimbursement, thereby unnecessarily using the costliest locus of care while creating insurmountable burdens on institutions treating AIDS patients.

Public hospitals in urban areas such as New York City, where the AIDS and low-income caseloads will continue to grow, would be forced to treat only the sickest patients or face a systemwide collapse as the demand for care comes to exceed available resources. Public institutions in restrictive Medicaid states such as Texas would find their local governments requiring them to absorb larger proportions of AIDS health care costs or to ration care. In states where Medicaid support has already been eroding, fewer and fewer providers would be able to accept people with AIDS, effectively dumping these individuals on public hospitals. As part of the tragic spiral, these institutions, in turn, would be faced with the choice of absorbing patients (and greater losses) or closing their doors.

Generally, there would be fewer initiatives and lower staff morale, and it is likely that community resentment toward expenditure of resources on AIDS patients would increase. The patchwork approach toward treating medically disenfranchised AIDS patients would accelerate the creation of the three-tier health care system described in Chapter 5.

Incremental change. Limited changes in AIDS health and health-related support could take many forms, with each alternative creating a number of potential outcomes. However, if incremental changes are implemented, they are likely to occur generally within established financing mechanisms and provider configurations.

In this scenario, the federal government provides financing that at least keeps pace with the major costs of hospital care for AIDS. Thus, Medicaid would continue to support low-income people with AIDS in some states. If states were encouraged to adopt changes in their minimal eligibility requirements—for example, by including some individuals whose health care expenses reduce them to poverty but who are not qualified to receive Medicaid—the Medicaid rolls could be expanded. Increases in minimal payments for inpatient services could keep some hospitals from excluding AIDS patients. In addition, Medicaid could provide low-income AIDS patients with a "buy-in" alternative, by which those who are above existing qualifying thresholds could pay to receive Medicaid benefits. Demonstration programs that encourage more cost effective and comprehensive treatment, or that target certain at-risk populations, would assist in establishing some progressive approaches to care.

Private payers could curtail their efforts to exclude people with AIDS. These insurers could also offer AIDS patients participation by creating expanded high-risk pools for uninsurable patients. Such an expansion would work by providing coverage for individuals with preexisting medical conditions that deny them insurance. If they are willing to pay higher premiums, they will be insured. Insurers, alone or in cooperation with states, would agree to underwrite their losses.

Communities with large numbers of AIDS sufferers could continue to provide support for the most urgently needed services. With support from public and private sources, it would be possible to expand noninpatient services modestly, allowing some growth in alternative types of care.

The impact of such changes on public hospitals, and on the overall care of people with AIDS, is likely to be minimal for a number of reasons. Efforts to keep pace with costs would most likely continue to focus on expensive inpatient care, simply because that is where financing and services are currently focused. Such initiatives would not address inequities in the provision of care, nor would they assist in reducing the evolving crises in public hospitals in New York City and other urban areas.

Efforts to encourage voluntary, state-level changes in Medicaid eligibility are also likely to meet with minimal and sporadic success. While some states might take advantage of incentives, others would be reluctant to increase their support substantially, due to historical precedent or financial constraints, unless required to do so. For example, southern states, historically reluctant to expand eligibility beyond the minimum, would probably not be inclined to take advantage of many options.

Federal and state programs to encourage high-risk individuals, or persons who are not qualified at present, to purchase insurance or to buy into Medicaid would also meet with minimal success. High-risk insurance pools usually set a premium that is well above individual standards. If people are unemployed, they are not likely to have the resources to pay such premiums or to direct spending to health care rather than daily necessities. Similarly, a buy-in program might attract some people, but near-poor and poor individuals would, in general, be very reluctant to expend their limited resources for such purposes.

Demonstration projects that finance care and provide out-of-hospital services would assist hospitals only marginally. Since they would likely be limited to a specific patient population, these initiatives would not address the bulk of the population in public hospitals. This leaves the question of how to treat HIV-infected individuals who are not diagnosed with AIDS.

Finally, this scenario does not encourage significant additional participation by private hospitals. There would be relatively little financial incentive for the private sector to become involved, since reimbursement would still be focused on costly inpatient care. In addition, lack of a coordinated, community-based approach would allow providers to act autonomously and increase the disparity between public and private sectors in the number and types of patients treated.

Fundamental and systemwide change. Major changes in AIDS care would address directly the immediate and most threatening problems facing people with AIDS and their health care providers: limited access to services, the unbalanced burden of care, fragmentation in the service system, interstate inequities in financing, and inadequate resources for care beyond the inpatient unit. There would also be a recognition of the longer-term realities: the rising number of people with AIDS, a growing reliance on public sector support, increasing demand for health and social support services, and higher costs. For far-reaching AIDS initiatives to be successful, they would need to enlist the support of communities and all levels of government. Such efforts would also consider eligibility, services, and financing for hospital, nonhospital, and other necessary care.

Communities affected by the AIDS epidemic would become an integral part of the planning for all the programs, coordinating services and continually monitoring the impact of the illness on their cities and counties. No one segment would assume responsibility. Instead, individual business leaders, chambers of commerce, local governmental representatives, service providers, community leaders, AIDS advocates, and volunteers would determine a course of action for all individuals, regardless of their ability to pay, and would be prepared to support or advocate essential and promising programs. States could encourage such activities by giving special funding consideration to coordinated efforts. They could also lend technical assistance to these communities.

Meanwhile, the federal government should assume responsibility for reducing the unevenness in Medicaid *eligibility* that now allows coverage in excess of 100 percent of the federal poverty level in some states and enables other states to set the qualifying limit at or below 25 percent of the poverty level. Phasing in coverage to 100 percent of poverty would reduce the current inequities. More importantly, elimination of severe state "spend-down" restrictions, which are so devastating for individuals forced to exhaust their available resources on medical expenses and for the providers who treat them, would assist greatly in qualifying many people with AIDS for Medicaid, relieving their financial pressures.

A primary goal of any service initiative would be to correct the large and growing imbalance in the provision of hospital care to people with AIDS. Federal, state, and local financial support for low-income AIDS patients through Medicaid or special programs, as well as community involvement, would be necessary but not sufficient. Both the public and private sectors must relieve the pressure on hospitals by supporting non-hospital-based services. For example, the federal government's home- and community-based waiver program allows states to develop out-of-hospital initiatives as alternatives to inpatient care only if the costs are not higher. Without encouraging profligate spending, the federal government, in cooperation with and monitored by states, could allow broader implementation of these alternatives at costs that are modestly higher than inpatient care if the programs meet rigorous additional criteria regarding scope of services and allocation of resources.

An existing federal program under the Department of Health and Human Services provides support for constructing and renovating structures for people with AIDS but receives little in appropriations. Increases in these funds could also be used to reduce the inpatient emphasis. The resources needed to provide care in skilled nursing facilities and other settings should be assessed in planning for alternative services. Finally, with regard to inpatient care, it may be necessary to apply community pressure or financial pressure through Medicaid reimbursements, or both, if certain hospitals clearly show that they are avoiding responsibility for AIDS inpatient care.

A comprehensive approach to caring for AIDS sufferers will require establishing a spectrum of services that is targeted to the needs of this population. The emphasis must shift away from the inpatient unit to make the community the service core. Such a continuum of care, with a focus on the areas we live in rather than the hospitals we use, would form the essence of any successful initiative.

Public and other hospitals serving large numbers of low-income people with AIDS have recognized a number of essential components to any continuum of care. Health experts insist, for example, that prevention and education are fundamental to halting the spread of this illness. Thus, any comprehensive approach to AIDS would include community-based efforts to identify and reach high-risk populations and the general citizenry. Programs must be targeted to the special circumstances of vulnerable groups. Minorities, particularly blacks, who are disproportionately affected, should be provided with information that takes into consideration their life-styles. IV drug users should have access to rehabilitation programs without waiting in line, as well as clean needles. Finally, testing on a voluntary basis should be widely available at low cost or for free.

For individuals requiring health services, community clinics and hospital outpatient departments would become the primary locus of care. These settings would serve two primary purposes. They would provide intervention early in a person's illness, keeping him or her at home or in a residence as long and as often as possible. They would also become focal points for health care and coordinating health related needs once the person enters more acute and debilitating stages of the illness.

The care available in these centers would extend far beyond basic services. To eliminate the pressure to receive treatment at inpatient units, these clinics would either include or have referral links to a wide array of interventions such as dental and mental health, oncology, dermatology, pharmaceutical resources, and pediatrics.

For the foreseeable future, however, it is inevitable that almost all people with AIDS will require inpatient care during the course of their illness. Treatment in a hospital setting would be reserved only for persons too ill to receive care elsewhere or for specialized care. It would not be necessary to establish an AIDS unit or designate a facility as an AIDS hospital. Instead, service configurations would be structured to provide the best fit with both the inpatient institution and the community. The comprehensive care program would also limit the inpatient stay to the minimal time necessary for treatment in that setting. Thus, the individual would return to the community as soon as it was practical to do so.

In addition to inpatient care, the course of this illness virtually guarantees that AIDS sufferers will require non-acute care assistance beyond what is provided in clinics. Some people will be able to function with minimal help, while others will need skilled care.

The ideal continuum of care would enable each patient to function in the least-restrictive setting. Programs would offer in-home nursing care, including drug therapy, as well as primary care and health-related services—housing, food, and basic living necessities. Intermediate care and skilled nursing facilities that are sensitive to the needs of people with AIDS would also be available. Specialized care for mental conditions would be part of the subacute services, as would hospice care for those who are in the terminal stage of the illness. The protocol for placement of these patients should also be sufficiently flexible so that patients could move easily within the various levels of acute and subacute care.

A large number of AIDS patients have no home or other setting to return to once they have received treatment. In particular, IV drug users, prostitutes, and the homeless may be left with no community-based residence. For people who do not require subacute care in an organized setting, residential facilities would be made available. These facilities would supervise medication, provide nutrition and other daily living necessities, and assure access to needed health services through a referral network.

With such an extensive array of available services and providers, it becomes vital to have a mechanism for systematic coordination and to keep inappropriate care to a minimum. To that end, an individual or a team would serve in a case-management capacity for each person with AIDS. Case managers would be responsible for assessing treatment protocols, linking individuals with appropriate care providers, evaluating the progress of treatment, and coordinating with representatives of health-related services. Case managers would also ensure that social services and other nonhealth services be provided as well as the health services component.

If any of the aforementioned proposals are to be realized, financing remains the crucial issue. Without question, such initiatives will require increased support from the federal government, but other sectors, both public and private, must be willing to accept responsibility as well.

Perhaps the most critical issue related to public hospital financing of AIDS treatment is ensuring fair and equitable coverage of inpatient and outpatient care. In lieu of national health insurance, states, in cooperation with the federal government, should guarantee a minimal level of Medicaid reimbursement throughout the United States to stem the erosion of providers who accept AIDS patients and to relieve the disproportionate burden on public hospitals. Outpatient Medicaid reimbursement, woefully inadequate for years, should also be revisited, first by assessing the national situation and then by taking action to correct glaring financial shortfalls. At the very least, Medicaid should compensate adequately outpatient hospital and clinic coverage for services that are clearly appropriate for people with AIDS. The role of the federal government in requiring expansion is especially critical for Medicaid, since politics may interfere with the enhancements proposed in many states.

It would be politically difficult to enact, but Congress and the administration should continue to consider the possibility of reducing or waiving the two-year waiting period for disabled AIDS patients to qualify for Medicare. Ironically, as AIDS becomes more of a chronic illness and treatments prolong the lives of people with AIDS, additional Medicare coverage will occur regardless of legislative action.

The impact on private insurance should also be assessed objectively. Where true threats to viability appear, all levels of government should develop stopgap programs to cap the losses the payers might incur. Otherwise, the private payers should be held accountable by states and localities for covering AIDS treatment costs without penalizing their beneficiaries.

Effective financing of a continuum of care or substantial parts thereof is more difficult. It must be structured with contributions from all levels of government. States, with their local governments, would take on additional responsibility for coordinating care (for example, through a core service agency) and assuring the existence of, and support for, essential service providers. Business and community leaders would recognize their role in assuring sufficient coverage and contributing to the financial base.

Under a more comprehensive approach to AIDS care, public hospitals in major cities would continue to serve residents in their communities and other AIDS patients who need their special tertiary services. However, the burden of AIDS care would be shared more equitably, not just with other hospitals but with many other local providers. In this manner, public hospitals would participate as essential service providers to all and not as a last refuge for the medically disenfranchised.

With a more enlightened program in place and with adequate financing, there would be fewer incentives to dump unwanted patients. Communitywide public and private sector monitoring of the epidemic's progress would help immeasurably in correcting health care imbalances and planning necessary next steps.

The concept of a successful continuum of care may seem too financially prohibitive for serious consideration. Yet, with basic support, some promising models have emerged with public hospitals at the core. Such initiatives, though small relative to the size of the epidemic, point out what is possible with sufficient support and attention. For example, the San Francisco Department of Public Health has been developing, expanding, and implementing a comprehensive plan whose goals are to educate the public and to screen individuals at high risk, to provide appropriate hospital treatment for people with AIDS, and to provide chronic care. This program model—which has used volunteers and obtained community support to meet the health, nutritional, social, and housing needs of people with AIDS—has been used nationwide.

Jackson Memorial Hospital in Miami is participating in the South Florida AIDS Network, which receives support from the state, the Robert Wood Johnson Foundation (RWJF), and the Health Resources and Services Administration (HRSA). The Network's goals are to provide care and treatment by "coordinating and mobilizing the community." The program is attempting to span the continuum of care and to work through a consortium of local social service and health agencies. New York City public hospitals and institutions in six other cities have developed similar programs with HRSA and RWJF support.

The New York City nonprofit hospitals are participating in a state-sponsored program that identifies certain facilities as AIDS centers. With assistance from New York State, these institutions agree to provide or coordinate all health services required by the AIDS patients they treat. The city's public hospitals are currently considering joining this program.

Conclusion

The health care needs of AIDS patients are not unique to this population. Indeed, they represent what is essential for so many who are uninsured and underserved in our society.

A focus on comprehensive care for AIDS patients may not be practical under our current health care system. Nor is it necessarily appropriate to single out this particular population when there are so many other poor and disadvantaged in desperate need. It is unlikely that the needs of disenfranchised AIDS patients and non-AIDS patients will be fulfilled until and unless we come to realize that a national health care effort that will address the needs of all Americans is required. One step on the road to developing such a national health care effort would be to adopt a short-term strategy of having local, state, and national leaders join together to encourage the distribution of the burden of care more equitably among all providers. If the idea of sharing the burden among public and private hospitals and between communities took hold, the road to national comprehensive care would be shortened. This would be the first step to some kind of national health care system, one that would address the needs of all citizens. Until then, any actions taken will only represent patchwork attempts that will serve to prolong the existence of a fragmented system.

There are many obstacles to progress. The national budget deficit looms largest and will be used, aptly or inappropriately, as an excuse for inaction. However, as we enter a new decade, we must decide how we, as a nation, will choose to use the lessons we have learned and are still learning from the current crisis. As we do so, we must remember that what we decide today will be seen tomorrow as a reflection of our humanity toward our fellow human beings.

Appendix
Two AIDS Surveys

In 1986, NAPH, together with the Association of American Medical Colleges' Council of Teaching Hospitals (COTH), released the 1985 Hospital AIDS Survey, funded by the Robert Wood Johnson Foundation. The purpose of the survey was to collect information on AIDS services in urban public and private teaching hospitals in 1985, including the types of patients treated, the array of services provided, and the costs and financing of those services. Hospitals belonging to these two associations were feeling the impact of the AIDS epidemic and hoped to assemble information on the nature and care of AIDS patients from the hospitals' perspective, something that had not previously been done at the national level. One hundred and ninety-eight hospitals, about 42 percent of the membership of the associations, responded. The information was compiled and has been widely cited to describe the impact of the AIDS epidemic on the hospital sector.

In order to monitor this situation over time, NAPH received funding from the Robert Wood Johnson Foundation and other sources to conduct a similar survey requesting information for 1987. For this survey, NAPH and COTH were joined by two other associations, the National Association of Children's Hospitals and Related Institutions (NACHRI), and the National Council of Community Hospitals (NCCH). Three hundred and forty-one hospitals responded to the 1987 survey, representing

55 percent of the membership of the four associations. The responses to these two surveys, particularly the responses of 55 NAPH members, are the basis for the tables and statistics throughout this book and those presented here.

Table 1
AIDS Patients in Public Hospitals in 1987, by Region

	Northeast	Midwest	South	West
Risk groups				
Homosexual	7%	65%	59%	72%
Homosexual/drug user	6	14	8	10
Heterosexual/drug user	67	13	12	11
Sex partner*	4	2	2	4
Child*	5	0	15	0
Blood product	1	6	5	2
Age				
0–2	3%	0%	8%	0%
3–19	1	1	3	0
20–49	90	94	84	94
50+	6	5	6	5
Sex				
Male	75%	93%	83%	96%
Female	25	7	17	4
Race				
Caucasian	13%	54%	43%	64%
Black	53	39	41	18
Hispanic	31	5	15	16
Other	2	2	1	2
Hospitals responding	**16**	**10**	**13**	**10**
Patients represented	**2848**	**287**	**1742**	**388**

* Of risk-group members.

Table 2
AIDS Patients' Utilization of Public Hospitals, by Region

	Northeast			Midwest		
	1985	1987	Change (%)	1985	1987	Change (%)
Patients						
Total	1,734	2,848	64	93	287	209
Average per hospital	116	178	53	12	29	142
Admissions						
Total	2,170	4,088	88	167	399	139
Average per hospital	145	256	77	21	40	90
Inpatient Days						
Total	58,174	97,181	67	2,559	5,758	125
Average per hospital	3,878	6,074	57	320	576	80
Average length of stay (in days)	26.8	23.8	− 11	15.3	14.4	− 6
Average number of days per patient per year	33.5	34.1	2	27.5	20.1	− 27
Average number of admissions per patient per year	1.3	1.4	8	1.8	1.4	− 22
Hospitals responding	**15**	**16**	**7**	**8**	**10**	**25**

Table 2
AIDS Patients' Utilization of Public Hospitals, by Region, continued

	South			West		
	1985	1987	Change (%)	1985	1987	Change (%)
Patients						
Total	415	1,742	320	735	1,216	65
Average per hospital	52	134	158	41	76	85
Admissions						
Total	621	2,438	293	1,309	2,191	67
Average per hospital	78	188	141	73	137	88
Inpatient days						
Total	10,549	33,531	218	19,812	29,566	49
Average per hospital	1,319	2,579	96	1,101	1,848	68
Average length of stay (in days)	17.0	13.8	-19	15.1	13.5	-11
Average number of days per patient per year	25.4	19.2	-24	27.0	24.3	-10
Average number of admissions per patient per year	1.5	1.4	-6	1.8	1.8	0
Hospitals responding	8	13	63	18	16	-11

Table 3

Level of Care for Inpatients with AIDS in Public Hospitals in 1987, Overall and by Region

	Total	Northeast	Midwest	South	West
Number of hospitals with designated AIDS units	7	3	0	3	1
Level of care					
ICU days	3%	3%	11%	2%	4%
Acute care days	89	86	83	96	96
Medically ready for discharge	8	11	6	2	0
Other days	0	0	0	0	0

Table 4
Discharge Disposition in 1987
(For AIDS Patients in Public Hospitals)

	%
Deaths	18
Home (no assistance)	47
Home (with assistance)	16
Long-term care	1
Intermediate care facility	0
Hospice	2
Acute care facility	1
Prison	1
Foster care	1
Other	13

Table 5
AIDS Patients' Use of Public Hospital Outpatient Services, Overall and by Region

	Total		Northeast		Midwest		South		West	
	1985	1987	1985	1987	1985	1987	1985	1987	1985	1987
Number of outpatient visits										
Total	18,338	50,797	1,505	12,134	340	3,645	718	21,681	15,775	13,337
Average per hospital	965	1,539	502	1,103	85	521	359	2,710	1,578	1,905
Number of outpatients										
Total	2,214	5,264	390	1,507	12	189	103	2,112	1,709	1,456
Average per hospital	130	170	130	137	3	27	51	264	171	208
Number of visits per patient	7	9	4	8	28	19	7	10	9	9
Hospitals responding	**19**	**33**	**3**	**11**	**4**	**7**	**2**	**8**	**10**	**7**

Table 6
Case Management and Links with Community Groups in 1987
(For Public Hospital AIDS Patients, in Percent of Respondents)

	Total	Northeast	Midwest	South	West
Hospitals with case management programs	46	79	40	33	29
Hospitals with links to groups representing					
Homosexuals	73	71	90	75	60
Drug users	60	85	60	42	53
Minorities	64	62	80	58	60
Women	52	69	20	58	53
Hemophiliacs	48	23	50	58	60
Adolescents	45	46	30	50	50
Parents with children at risk	54	69	11	67	57
Number of hospitals responding	**55**	**16**	**10**	**13**	**16**

Table 7
Payer Sources Overall and by Region
(For Inpatients with AIDS in Public Hospitals, by Percent)

	Total		Northeast		Midwest		South		West	
	1985	1987	1985	1987	1985	1987	1985	1987	1985	1987
Payer source										
Medicare	1	2	1	2	5	0	2	1	2	3
Medicaid	62	54	69	72	57	53	16	18	60	62
Selfpay and other	25	33	18	13	13	34	74	68	26	27
Private insurance	8	9	6	9	23	11	6	11	11	8
Prisoner	4	2	6	4	1	2	2	2	1	0

Table 8
Outpatient Payer Sources in 1987
(For AIDS Patients in Public Hospitals*)

	%
Medicare	2
Medicaid	24
Selfpay and other	64
Private insurance	10
Prisoner	0

* Based on 18 hospitals and 27,184 visits.

Table 9
Outpatient Costs and Revenues in 1987
(For AIDS Patients and Others in Public Hospitals*)

Costs and revenues for AIDS patients
    Cost per visit $ 159
    Cost per patient per year   1,749

    Revenue per visit   41
    Revenue per patient per year   451

    Loss per visit   118
    Loss per patient per year   1,298

Costs and revenue for other outpatients
    Cost per visit   105
    Revenue per visit   51
    Loss per visit   54

* Based on 19 hospitals.

Figure 1
NAPH Membership: Net Revenue 1985
(40 Member Hospitals)

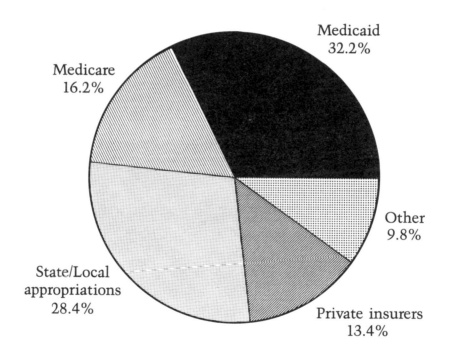

Total net revenue of $6 billion

Figure 2
Specialized Services Provided by Public and
Other Short-Term General Hospitals

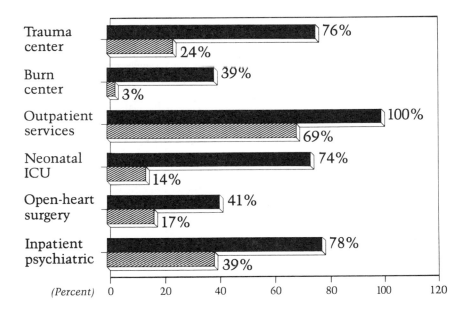

NAPH Hospitals

Other Hospitals

Trauma center — 76% / 24%
Burn center — 39% / 3%
Outpatient services — 100% / 69%
Neonatal ICU — 74% / 14%
Open-heart surgery — 41% / 17%
Inpatient psychiatric — 78% / 39%

(Percent) 0 20 40 60 80 100 120

Source: This material is based on the 1987 *American Hospital Association Guide* as well as NAPH figures.

Notes

Chapter 2

1. E. Friedman, "Public Hospitals: Doing What Everyone Wants Done but Few Others Wish to Do," *Journal of the American Medical Association* 257, no. 11 (March 20, 1987). See also L. S. Gage, D. P. Andrulis, and V. Beers, *America's Health Safety Net: A Report on the Situation of Public Hospitals in Our Nation's Metropolitan Areas* (Washington, D.C.: National Association of Public Hospitals, 1987).

2. J. Hadley and J. Feder, *Hospitals' Care to the Poor in 1980* (Washington, D.C.: The Urban Institute, 1983).

3. J. Feder, J. Hadley, and R. Mullner, *Falling Through the Cracks: Poverty, Insurance Coverage and Hospitals' Care to the Poor, 1980 and 1982.* (Washington, D.C.: The Urban Institute, 1984).

4. *America's Health Safety Net*, 1987.

5. V. Beers Weslowski, National Association of Public Hospitals, personal communication with the author, Washington, D.C., 1989.

6. "Emergency Rooms Overwhelmed as New York's Poor Get Sicker," *The New York Times*, December 19, 1988.

7. *America's Health Safety Net*, 1987.

Chapter 3

1. Ford Foundation, *The Common Good: Social Welfare and the American Future* (New York: The Ford Foundation, 1989), p. 57.

2. Friedman, "Public Hospitals," pp. 3-4.

3. *America's Health Safety Net*, 1987, p. 13.

4. National Association of Public Hospitals, "The Situation of the Nation's Urban Public Hospitals," unpublished report, 1989.

5. Friedman, "Public Hospitals," p. 5.

6. Ibid.

7. E. Friedman, "Public Hospitals Often Face Unmet Capital Needs, Underfunding, Uncompensated Patient Care Costs," *Journal of the American Medical Association* 257, no. 14 (April 10, 1987), p. 11.

8. L. S. Gage, statement before the House Ways and Means Committee, March 1, 1989.

9. Ibid., p. 7.

10. David Ramsay, statement before the Senate Committee on Labor and Human Resources, May 1, 1989.

11. K. Fireman, "A System Out of Balance," *New York Newsday*, May 4, 1989, p. 8.

12. Ibid.

13. Ibid., p. 35.

Chapter 4

1. Centers for Disease Control, *Weekly Surveillance Report*, December 26, 1988.

2. *The AIDS/HIV Record*, Resource Supplement 2:23 (December 1988).

3. Panos Institute, *AIDS and the Third World*, Panos Dossier 1 (Washington, D.C.: November 1988).

4. T. Quinn, F. Zacarias, R. St. John, "AIDS in the Americas," *New England Journal of Medicine* 320, no. 15 (April 13, 1989): 1105-7

5. A. Scitovsky and D. Rice, "Estimates of the Direct and Indirect Costs of Acquired Immune Deficiency Syndrome," *Public Health Report* 102 (1987): 1-17.

6. A. Scitovsky, "The Economic Impact of AIDS in the United States," *Health Affairs* 7, no. 4 (Fall 1988): 32-45.

7. Centers for Disease Control, *Weekly Surveillance Report*, December 26, 1988.

8. D. Andrulis et al., "The Provision and Financing of Medical Care for AIDS Patients in US Public and Private Teaching Hospitals," *Journal of the American Medical Association* 258, no. 10 (September 11, 1987): 1343-46.

9. P. Arno and R. Hughes, "Local Policy Responses to the AIDS Epidemic: New York, San Francisco," *New York State Journal of Medicine* 87 (1987): 264-72.

10. Andrulis, "Provision and Financing of Medical Care," pp. 1343-46.

11. "Health Resources and Services Administration," unpublished summary from meeting on Non-Acute Care Facilities for AIDS, Rockville, Md., March 2, 1988.

12. Andrulis, "Provision and Financing of Medical Care," pp. 1343-46.

13. Health Care Financing Program Statistics, *Medicare and Medicaid Data Book, 1984,* HCFA pub. no. 03210 (1986).

14. "News Summaries," *AIDS Policy and Law* (Washington, D.C.: Buraff Publications, November 30, 1988).

15. J. Kelly, J. Ball, and B. Turner, "Severity of Illness in Use of Hospital Resources by AIDS Patients," paper presented at the Fourth International Conference on AIDS, Stockholm, June 1988.

16. *Local Area AIDS Data,* Claritas Corporation, Alexandria, Va., July, 1988.

Chapter 5

1. President's Commission on the HIV Epidemic, hearings on Care of HIV-infected Persons, Washington, D.C., January 13-15, 1988.

2. Statement by Congressman Pete Stark, *Congressional Record,* September 9, 1988, p. E2850.

3. R. Ratzan and H. Schneiderman, "AIDS, Autopsies and Abandonment," *Journal of the American Medical Association* 260, no. 23 (December 16, 1988): 3466-69.

4. D. Andrulis and V. Beers, "Coordinating Hospital and Community-based Care for AIDS Patients," *Journal of Ambulatory Care Management* 11, no. 2 (1988): 5-13.

5. P. Moore, "AIDS: The New York City Public Hospital Ex-

perience," paper presented at the Second National AIDS Conference, San Francisco, September 30, 1988.

Chapter 6

1. H. Dowling, *City Hospitals* (Cambridge, Mass.: Harvard University Press, 1982).

2. Report of the Presidential Commission on the Human Immunodeficiency Virus Epidemic, Washington, D.C., June 24, 1988.

Index